# INTRODUCING

*Little Fighters*

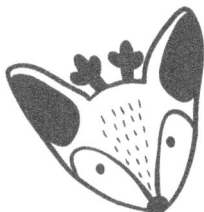

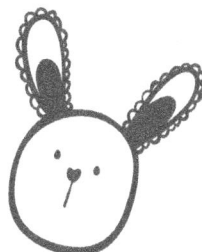

_____
Name

BORN ON ........................................

THE ............ DAY OF ....................

IN THE YEAR ............ .

@TIME

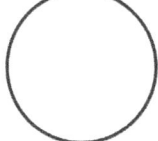

pounds / ounces

DOCTOR ........................................

Hospital

_____
Name

BORN ON ........................................

THE ............ DAY OF ....................

IN THE YEAR ............ .

@TIME

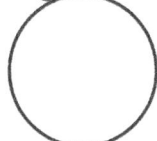

pounds / ounces

DOCTOR ........................................

Hospital

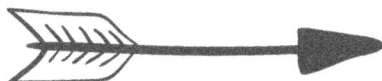

YOU ARE MY HAPPY

# VISITORS

*Please Sign In*

| DATE | NAME / NOTE |
|------|-------------|
|      |             |
|      |             |
|      |             |
|      |             |
|      |             |
|      |             |
|      |             |
|      |             |
|      |             |
|      |             |
|      |             |
|      |             |
|      |             |
|      |             |

DATE

NAME / NOTE

# SMALL BUT MIGHTY

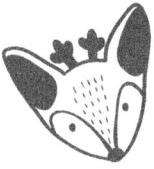
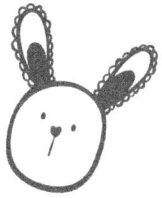

DATE:

_____
NAME

_____
NAME

○ NICU DAY # ____
○ HOME DAY # ____

GESTATIONAL AGE:

WEIGHT:

GESTATIONAL AGE:

WEIGHT:

○ NICU DAY # ____
○ HOME DAY # ____

## Today We Got To

☐ PHONE CALL    ☐ SKIN TO SKIN    ☐ SING
☐ TOUCH         ☐ TAKE TEMP       ☐ BATH
☐ DIAPER        ☐ FEEDING         ☐ MASSAGE
☐ HOLD          ☐ READ            ☐ VISITORS

☐ PHONE CALL    ☐ SKIN TO SKIN    ☐ SING
☐ TOUCH         ☐ TAKE TEMP       ☐ BATH
☐ DIAPER        ☐ FEEDING         ☐ MASSAGE
☐ HOLD          ☐ READ            ☐ VISITORS

## Feedings

_____     _____
_____     _____
_____     _____
_____     _____
_____     _____
_____     _____
_____     _____
_____     _____

## Medical Stats

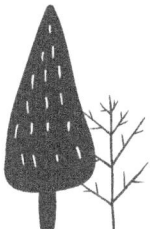
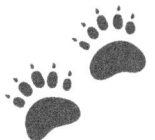

# Journaling

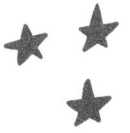

_____
_____
_____
_____
_____
_____
_____
_____
_____
_____
_____
_____
_____
_____

## QUESTIONS
TO ASK

_____
_____
_____
_____

Today I'm Grateful For...

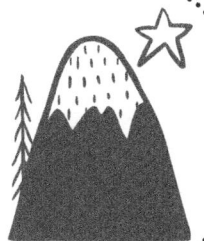

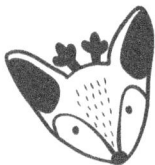

DATE:

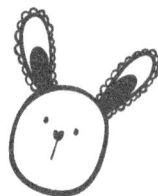

_____
NAME

_____
NAME

○ NICU DAY # ____
○ HOME DAY # ____

GESTATIONAL AGE:

WEIGHT:

GESTATIONAL AGE:

WEIGHT:

○ NICU DAY # ____
○ HOME DAY # ____

## Today We Got To

☐ PHONE CALL  ☐ SKIN TO SKIN  ☐ SING
☐ TOUCH       ☐ TAKE TEMP     ☐ BATH
☐ DIAPER      ☐ FEEDING       ☐ MASSAGE
☐ HOLD        ☐ READ          ☐ VISITORS

☐ PHONE CALL  ☐ SKIN TO SKIN  ☐ SING
☐ TOUCH       ☐ TAKE TEMP     ☐ BATH
☐ DIAPER      ☐ FEEDING       ☐ MASSAGE
☐ HOLD        ☐ READ          ☐ VISITORS

## Feedings

_____
_____
_____
_____
_____
_____
_____
_____

_____
_____
_____
_____
_____
_____
_____
_____

## Medical Stats

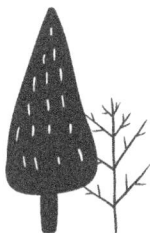

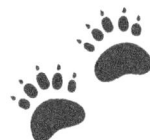

# Journaling

QUESTIONS
TO ASK

Today I'm Grateful For...

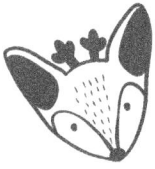
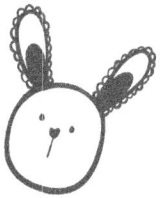

DATE:

_____          _____
NAME                                      NAME

○ NICU DAY # ____   ┌─────────────────┐   ┌─────────────────┐   ○ NICU DAY # ____
○ HOME DAY # ____   │ GESTATIONAL AGE: │   │ GESTATIONAL AGE: │   ○ HOME DAY # ____
                    │ WEIGHT:          │   │ WEIGHT:          │

## Today We Got To

□ PHONE CALL    □ SKIN TO SKIN    □ SING       □ PHONE CALL    □ SKIN TO SKIN    □ SING
□ TOUCH         □ TAKE TEMP       □ BATH       □ TOUCH         □ TAKE TEMP       □ BATH
□ DIAPER        □ FEEDING         □ MASSAGE    □ DIAPER        □ FEEDING         □ MASSAGE
□ HOLD          □ READ            □ VISITORS   □ HOLD          □ READ            □ VISITORS

## Feedings

_____          _____
_____          _____
_____          _____
_____          _____
_____          _____
_____          _____
_____          _____
_____          _____

## Medical Stats

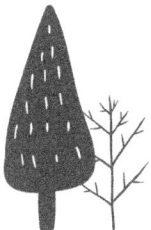
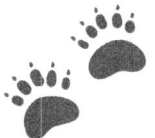

# Journaling

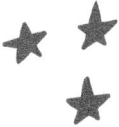

**QUESTIONS**
TO ASK

Today I'm Grateful For...

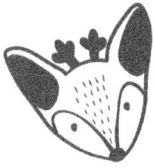
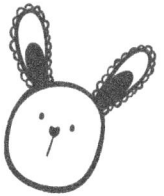

| DATE: |
|---|

_____  _____
NAME                                              NAME

○ NICU DAY # ____          GESTATIONAL AGE:          GESTATIONAL AGE:          ○ NICU DAY # ____
○ HOME DAY # ____          WEIGHT:          WEIGHT:          ○ HOME DAY # ____

## Today We Got To

☐ PHONE CALL  ☐ SKIN TO SKIN  ☐ SING          ☐ PHONE CALL  ☐ SKIN TO SKIN  ☐ SING
☐ TOUCH            ☐ TAKE TEMP       ☐ BATH          ☐ TOUCH            ☐ TAKE TEMP       ☐ BATH
☐ DIAPER          ☐ FEEDING            ☐ MASSAGE   ☐ DIAPER          ☐ FEEDING            ☐ MASSAGE
☐ HOLD              ☐ READ                  ☐ VISITORS    ☐ HOLD              ☐ READ                  ☐ VISITORS

## Feedings

_____          _____
_____          _____
_____          _____
_____          _____
_____          _____
_____          _____
_____          _____
_____          _____

## Medical Stats

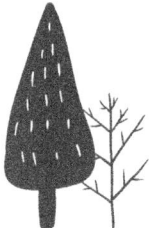
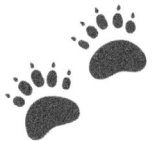

# Journaling

_____

_____

_____

_____

_____

_____

_____

_____

_____

_____

_____

_____

_____

## QUESTIONS
TO ASK

_____

_____

_____

_____

_____

_____

Today I'm Grateful For...

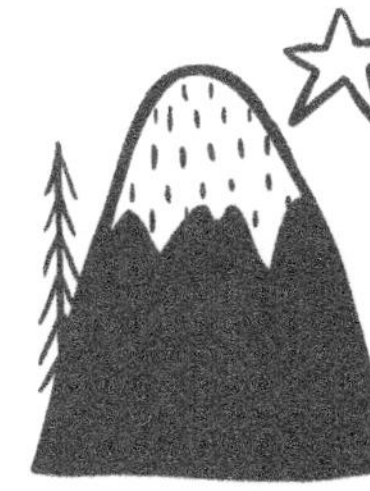

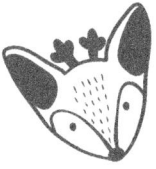
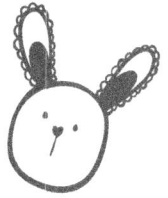

| DATE: |
|---|

_____ NAME

_____ NAME

○ NICU DAY # ____
○ HOME DAY # ____

| GESTATIONAL AGE: |
| WEIGHT: |

| GESTATIONAL AGE: |
| WEIGHT: |

○ NICU DAY # ____
○ HOME DAY # ____

## Today We Got To

☐ PHONE CALL
☐ TOUCH
☐ DIAPER
☐ HOLD

☐ SKIN TO SKIN
☐ TAKE TEMP
☐ FEEDING
☐ READ

☐ SING
☐ BATH
☐ MASSAGE
☐ VISITORS

☐ PHONE CALL
☐ TOUCH
☐ DIAPER
☐ HOLD

☐ SKIN TO SKIN
☐ TAKE TEMP
☐ FEEDING
☐ READ

☐ SING
☐ BATH
☐ MASSAGE
☐ VISITORS

## Feedings

_____
_____
_____
_____
_____
_____
_____
_____
_____

_____
_____
_____
_____
_____
_____
_____
_____
_____

## Medical Stats

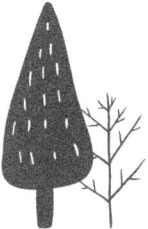
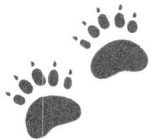

# Journaling

_____
_____
_____
_____
_____
_____
_____
_____
_____
_____
_____
_____
_____
_____
_____
_____
_____
_____
_____

## QUESTIONS
TO ASK

Today I'm Grateful For...

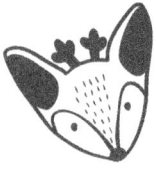
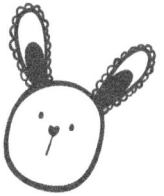

DATE:

_____  _____
NAME                                              NAME

○ NICU DAY # ____    GESTATIONAL AGE:          GESTATIONAL AGE:          ○ NICU DAY # ____
○ HOME DAY # ____    WEIGHT:                    WEIGHT:                    ○ HOME DAY # ____

## Today We Got To

☐ PHONE CALL    ☐ SKIN TO SKIN    ☐ SING        ☐ PHONE CALL    ☐ SKIN TO SKIN    ☐ SING
☐ TOUCH         ☐ TAKE TEMP       ☐ BATH        ☐ TOUCH         ☐ TAKE TEMP       ☐ BATH
☐ DIAPER        ☐ FEEDING         ☐ MASSAGE     ☐ DIAPER        ☐ FEEDING         ☐ MASSAGE
☐ HOLD          ☐ READ            ☐ VISITORS    ☐ HOLD          ☐ READ            ☐ VISITORS

## Feedings

_____          _____
_____          _____
_____          _____
_____          _____
_____          _____
_____          _____
_____          _____
_____          _____

## Medical Stats

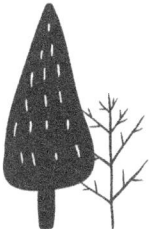
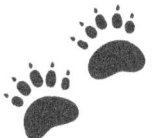

# Journaling

_____
_____
_____
_____
_____
_____
_____
_____
_____
_____
_____
_____
_____
_____
_____
_____
_____
_____
_____
_____

QUESTIONS
TO ASK

Today I'm Grateful For...

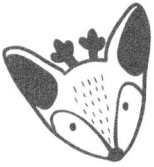
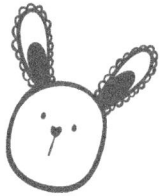

DATE:

_____          _____
NAME                                NAME

○ NICU DAY # ____    GESTATIONAL AGE:      GESTATIONAL AGE:    ○ NICU DAY # ____
○ HOME DAY # ____    WEIGHT:               WEIGHT:             ○ HOME DAY # ____

## Today We Got To

☐ PHONE CALL    ☐ SKIN TO SKIN    ☐ SING       ☐ PHONE CALL    ☐ SKIN TO SKIN    ☐ SING
☐ TOUCH         ☐ TAKE TEMP       ☐ BATH       ☐ TOUCH         ☐ TAKE TEMP       ☐ BATH
☐ DIAPER        ☐ FEEDING         ☐ MASSAGE    ☐ DIAPER        ☐ FEEDING         ☐ MASSAGE
☐ HOLD          ☐ READ            ☐ VISITORS   ☐ HOLD          ☐ READ            ☐ VISITORS

## Feedings

_____          _____
_____          _____
_____          _____
_____          _____
_____          _____
_____          _____
_____          _____
_____          _____

## Medical Stats

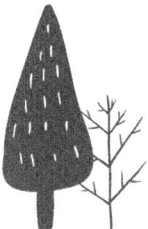
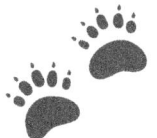

# Journaling

_____
_____
_____
_____
_____
_____
_____
_____
_____
_____
_____
_____
_____
_____
_____
_____

## QUESTIONS
TO ASK

Today I'm Grateful For...

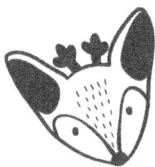
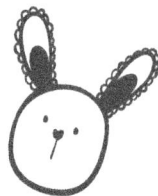

DATE:

_____
NAME

_____
NAME

○ NICU DAY # ____
○ HOME DAY # ____

GESTATIONAL AGE:

WEIGHT:

GESTATIONAL AGE:

WEIGHT:

○ NICU DAY # ____
○ HOME DAY # ____

## Today We Got To

☐ PHONE CALL  ☐ SKIN TO SKIN  ☐ SING
☐ TOUCH  ☐ TAKE TEMP  ☐ BATH
☐ DIAPER  ☐ FEEDING  ☐ MASSAGE
☐ HOLD  ☐ READ  ☐ VISITORS

☐ PHONE CALL  ☐ SKIN TO SKIN  ☐ SING
☐ TOUCH  ☐ TAKE TEMP  ☐ BATH
☐ DIAPER  ☐ FEEDING  ☐ MASSAGE
☐ HOLD  ☐ READ  ☐ VISITORS

## Feedings

_____
_____
_____
_____
_____
_____
_____
_____

_____
_____
_____
_____
_____
_____
_____
_____

## Medical Stats

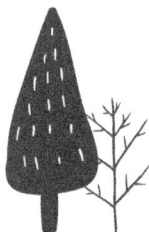
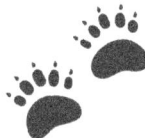

# Journaling

_____
_____
_____
_____
_____
_____
_____
_____
_____
_____
_____
_____
_____
_____
_____
_____
_____
_____
_____

## QUESTIONS
TO ASK

## Today I'm Grateful For...

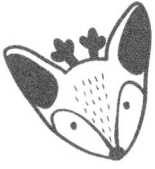
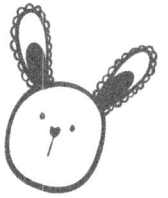

DATE: _____

_____                    _____
NAME                                    NAME

○ NICU DAY # ____     GESTATIONAL AGE:        GESTATIONAL AGE:        ○ NICU DAY # ____
○ HOME DAY # ____     WEIGHT:                 WEIGHT:                 ○ HOME DAY # ____

## Today We Got To

| ☐ PHONE CALL | ☐ SKIN TO SKIN | ☐ SING | ☐ PHONE CALL | ☐ SKIN TO SKIN | ☐ SING |
| ☐ TOUCH | ☐ TAKE TEMP | ☐ BATH | ☐ TOUCH | ☐ TAKE TEMP | ☐ BATH |
| ☐ DIAPER | ☐ FEEDING | ☐ MASSAGE | ☐ DIAPER | ☐ FEEDING | ☐ MASSAGE |
| ☐ HOLD | ☐ READ | ☐ VISITORS | ☐ HOLD | ☐ READ | ☐ VISITORS |

## Feedings

_____        _____
_____        _____
_____        _____
_____        _____
_____        _____
_____        _____
_____        _____
_____        _____

## Medical Stats

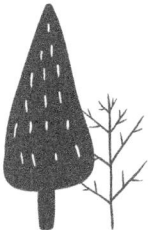
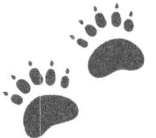

# Journaling

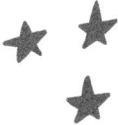

_____
_____
_____
_____
_____
_____
_____
_____
_____
_____
_____
_____
_____
_____

### QUESTIONS
TO ASK

_____
_____
_____
_____

Today I'm Grateful For...

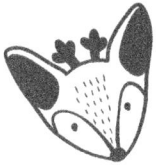
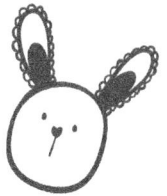

DATE:

_____ NAME

_____ NAME

○ NICU DAY # ____
○ HOME DAY # ____

GESTATIONAL AGE:

WEIGHT:

GESTATIONAL AGE:

WEIGHT:

○ NICU DAY # ____
○ HOME DAY # ____

## Today We Got To

☐ PHONE CALL   ☐ SKIN TO SKIN   ☐ SING
☐ TOUCH        ☐ TAKE TEMP      ☐ BATH
☐ DIAPER       ☐ FEEDING        ☐ MASSAGE
☐ HOLD         ☐ READ           ☐ VISITORS

☐ PHONE CALL   ☐ SKIN TO SKIN   ☐ SING
☐ TOUCH        ☐ TAKE TEMP      ☐ BATH
☐ DIAPER       ☐ FEEDING        ☐ MASSAGE
☐ HOLD         ☐ READ           ☐ VISITORS

## Feedings

_____
_____
_____
_____
_____
_____
_____
_____
_____

_____
_____
_____
_____
_____
_____
_____
_____
_____

## Medical Stats

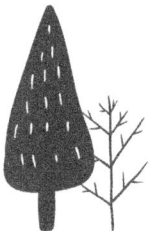
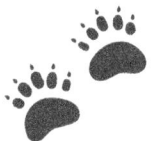

# Journaling

QUESTIONS
TO ASK

Today I'm Grateful For...

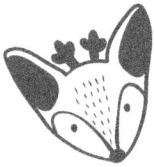
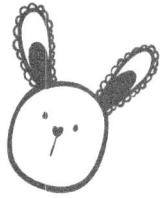

DATE:

_____          _____
NAME                                                    NAME

○ NICU DAY # ____          GESTATIONAL AGE:          GESTATIONAL AGE:          ○ NICU DAY # ____
○ HOME DAY # ____         WEIGHT:                              WEIGHT:                         ○ HOME DAY # ____

## Today We Got To

☐ PHONE CALL    ☐ SKIN TO SKIN    ☐ SING          ☐ PHONE CALL    ☐ SKIN TO SKIN    ☐ SING
☐ TOUCH               ☐ TAKE TEMP       ☐ BATH        ☐ TOUCH               ☐ TAKE TEMP       ☐ BATH
☐ DIAPER             ☐ FEEDING            ☐ MASSAGE   ☐ DIAPER             ☐ FEEDING            ☐ MASSAGE
☐ HOLD                 ☐ READ                  ☐ VISITORS    ☐ HOLD                 ☐ READ                  ☐ VISITORS

## Feedings

_____          _____
_____          _____
_____          _____
_____          _____
_____          _____
_____          _____
_____          _____
_____          _____

## Medical Stats

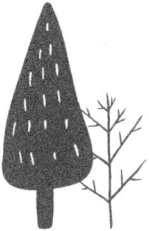
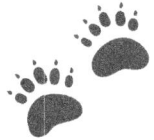

# Journaling

_____

_____

_____

_____

_____

_____

_____

_____

_____

_____

_____

_____

_____

_____

_____

## QUESTIONS
### TO ASK

_____

_____

_____

_____

Today I'm Grateful For...

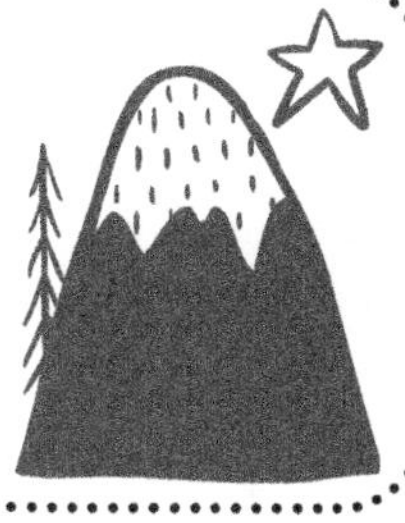

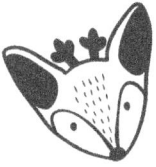
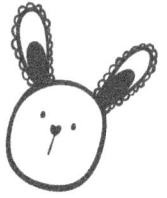

## DATE:

_____  
NAME

_____  
NAME

○ NICU DAY # ____  
○ HOME DAY # ____

GESTATIONAL AGE:  
WEIGHT:

GESTATIONAL AGE:  
WEIGHT:

○ NICU DAY # ____  
○ HOME DAY # ____

## Today We Got To

☐ PHONE CALL ☐ SKIN TO SKIN ☐ SING  
☐ TOUCH ☐ TAKE TEMP ☐ BATH  
☐ DIAPER ☐ FEEDING ☐ MASSAGE  
☐ HOLD ☐ READ ☐ VISITORS

☐ PHONE CALL ☐ SKIN TO SKIN ☐ SING  
☐ TOUCH ☐ TAKE TEMP ☐ BATH  
☐ DIAPER ☐ FEEDING ☐ MASSAGE  
☐ HOLD ☐ READ ☐ VISITORS

## Feedings

_____  
_____  
_____  
_____  
_____  
_____  
_____  
_____  
_____

_____  
_____  
_____  
_____  
_____  
_____  
_____  
_____  
_____

## Medical Stats

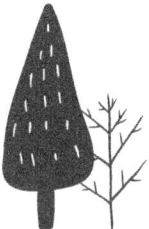
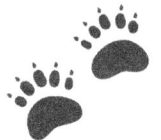

# Journaling

_____
_____
_____
_____
_____
_____
_____
_____
_____
_____
_____
_____
_____
_____
_____
_____
_____
_____

## QUESTIONS
TO ASK

Today I'm Grateful For...

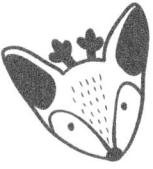
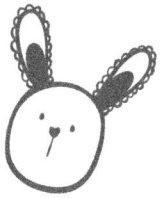

DATE:

_____                    _____
NAME                                          NAME

○ NICU DAY # ____    GESTATIONAL AGE:         GESTATIONAL AGE:        ○ NICU DAY # ____
○ HOME DAY # ____    WEIGHT:                  WEIGHT:                 ○ HOME DAY # ____

## Today We Got To

□ PHONE CALL   □ SKIN TO SKIN   □ SING      □ PHONE CALL   □ SKIN TO SKIN   □ SING
□ TOUCH        □ TAKE TEMP      □ BATH      □ TOUCH        □ TAKE TEMP      □ BATH
□ DIAPER       □ FEEDING        □ MASSAGE   □ DIAPER       □ FEEDING        □ MASSAGE
□ HOLD         □ READ           □ VISITORS  □ HOLD         □ READ           □ VISITORS

## Feedings

_____                    _____
_____                    _____
_____                    _____
_____                    _____
_____                    _____
_____                    _____
_____                    _____
_____                    _____

## Medical Stats

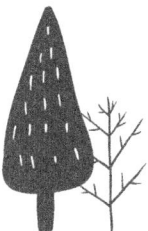
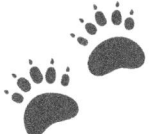

# Journaling

_____

_____

_____

_____

_____

_____

_____

_____

_____

_____

_____

_____

_____

## QUESTIONS
### TO ASK

_____

_____

_____

_____

Today I'm Grateful For...

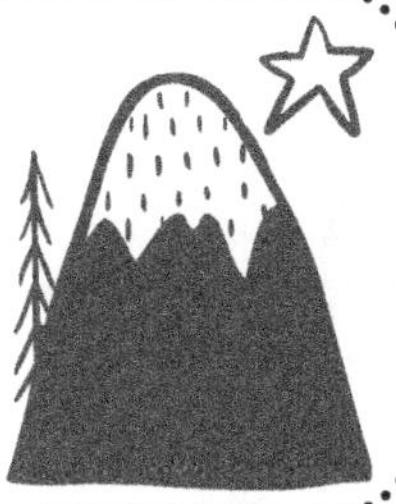

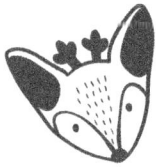
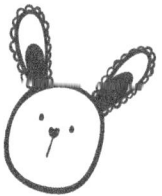

DATE

_____ NAME          _____ NAME

○ NICU DAY # ____    GESTATIONAL AGE:        GESTATIONAL AGE:        ○ NICU DAY # ____
○ HOME DAY # ____    WEIGHT:                 WEIGHT:                 ○ HOME DAY # ____

## Today We Got To

☐ PHONE CALL    ☐ SKIN TO SKIN    ☐ SING        ☐ PHONE CALL    ☐ SKIN TO SKIN    ☐ SING
☐ TOUCH         ☐ TAKE TEMP       ☐ BATH        ☐ TOUCH         ☐ TAKE TEMP       ☐ BATH
☐ DIAPER        ☐ FEEDING         ☐ MASSAGE     ☐ DIAPER        ☐ FEEDING         ☐ MASSAGE
☐ HOLD          ☐ READ            ☐ VISITORS    ☐ HOLD          ☐ READ            ☐ VISITORS

## Feedings

_____          _____
_____          _____
_____          _____
_____          _____
_____          _____
_____          _____
_____          _____
_____          _____
_____          _____

## Medical Stats

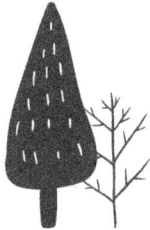
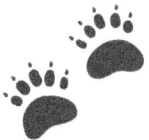

# Journaling

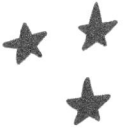

_____

_____

_____

_____

_____

_____

_____

_____

_____

_____

_____

_____

_____

_____

_____

_____

_____

_____

## QUESTIONS
TO ASK

## Today I'm Grateful For...

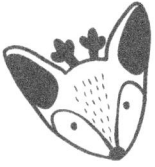
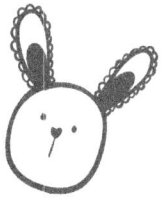

**DATE:**

_____ NAME

_____ NAME

○ NICU DAY # ____
○ HOME DAY # ____

GESTATIONAL AGE:

WEIGHT:

GESTATIONAL AGE:

WEIGHT:

○ NICU DAY # ____
○ HOME DAY # ____

## Today We Got To

☐ PHONE CALL
☐ TOUCH
☐ DIAPER
☐ HOLD

☐ SKIN TO SKIN
☐ TAKE TEMP
☐ FEEDING
☐ READ

☐ SING
☐ BATH
☐ MASSAGE
☐ VISITORS

☐ PHONE CALL
☐ TOUCH
☐ DIAPER
☐ HOLD

☐ SKIN TO SKIN
☐ TAKE TEMP
☐ FEEDING
☐ READ

☐ SING
☐ BATH
☐ MASSAGE
☐ VISITORS

## Feedings

_____
_____
_____
_____
_____
_____
_____
_____

_____
_____
_____
_____
_____
_____
_____
_____

## Medical Stats

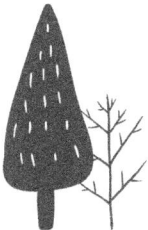
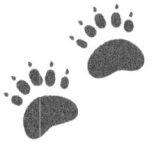

# Journaling

QUESTIONS
TO ASK

Today I'm Grateful For...

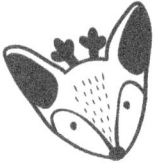
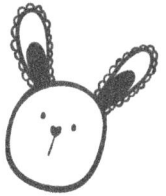

DATE:

_____          _____
NAME                                          NAME

○ NICU DAY # ____    GESTATIONAL AGE:        GESTATIONAL AGE:        ○ NICU DAY # ____
○ HOME DAY # ____    WEIGHT:                 WEIGHT:                 ○ HOME DAY # ____

## Today We Got To

☐ PHONE CALL    ☐ SKIN TO SKIN    ☐ SING       ☐ PHONE CALL    ☐ SKIN TO SKIN    ☐ SING
☐ TOUCH         ☐ TAKE TEMP       ☐ BATH       ☐ TOUCH         ☐ TAKE TEMP       ☐ BATH
☐ DIAPER        ☐ FEEDING         ☐ MASSAGE    ☐ DIAPER        ☐ FEEDING         ☐ MASSAGE
☐ HOLD          ☐ READ            ☐ VISITORS   ☐ HOLD          ☐ READ            ☐ VISITORS

## Feedings

_____          _____
_____          _____
_____          _____
_____          _____
_____          _____
_____          _____
_____          _____
_____          _____

## Medical Stats

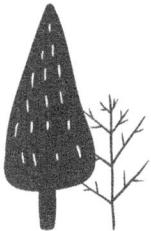
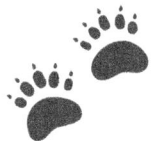

# Journaling

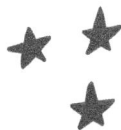

_____
_____
_____
_____
_____
_____
_____
_____
_____
_____
_____
_____
_____
_____
_____

## QUESTIONS
TO ASK

_____
_____
_____
_____

Today I'm Grateful For...

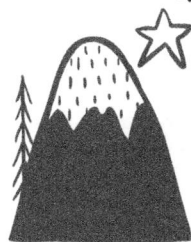

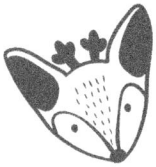
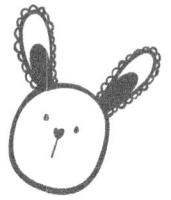

## DATE:

_____
NAME

_____
NAME

○ NICU DAY # ____
○ HOME DAY # ____

GESTATIONAL AGE:

WEIGHT:

GESTATIONAL AGE:

WEIGHT:

○ NICU DAY # ____
○ HOME DAY # ____

### Today We Got To

☐ PHONE CALL   ☐ SKIN TO SKIN   ☐ SING
☐ TOUCH        ☐ TAKE TEMP      ☐ BATH
☐ DIAPER       ☐ FEEDING        ☐ MASSAGE
☐ HOLD         ☐ READ           ☐ VISITORS

☐ PHONE CALL   ☐ SKIN TO SKIN   ☐ SING
☐ TOUCH        ☐ TAKE TEMP      ☐ BATH
☐ DIAPER       ☐ FEEDING        ☐ MASSAGE
☐ HOLD         ☐ READ           ☐ VISITORS

### Feedings

_____          _____
_____          _____
_____          _____
_____          _____
_____          _____
_____          _____
_____          _____
_____          _____

### Medical Stats

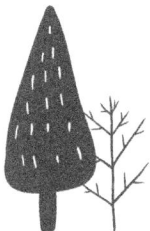
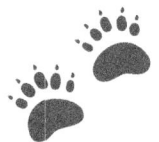

Journaling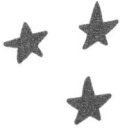

_____
_____
_____
_____
_____
_____
_____
_____
_____
_____
_____
_____
_____

QUESTIONS
TO ASK

_____
_____
_____
_____
_____

Today I'm Grateful For...

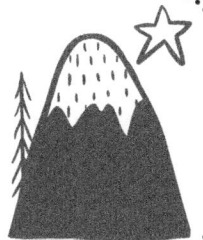

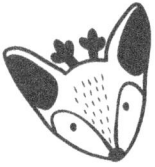
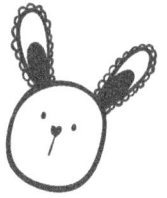

DATE:

NAME

NAME

○ NICU DAY # ____
○ HOME DAY # ____

GESTATIONAL AGE:

WEIGHT:

GESTATIONAL AGE:

WEIGHT:

○ NICU DAY # ____
○ HOME DAY # ____

## Today We Got To

☐ PHONE CALL    ☐ SKIN TO SKIN    ☐ SING
☐ TOUCH         ☐ TAKE TEMP       ☐ BATH
☐ DIAPER        ☐ FEEDING         ☐ MASSAGE
☐ HOLD          ☐ READ            ☐ VISITORS

☐ PHONE CALL    ☐ SKIN TO SKIN    ☐ SING
☐ TOUCH         ☐ TAKE TEMP       ☐ BATH
☐ DIAPER        ☐ FEEDING         ☐ MASSAGE
☐ HOLD          ☐ READ            ☐ VISITORS

## Feedings

## Medical Stats

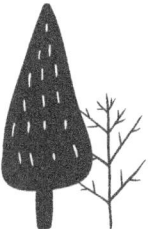
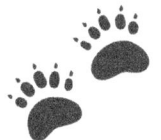

# Journaling

QUESTIONS
TO ASK

Today I'm Grateful For...

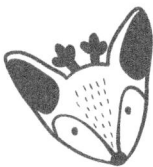
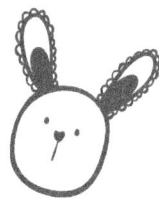

DATE:

_____    _____
NAME                           NAME

○ NICU DAY # ____    GESTATIONAL AGE:         GESTATIONAL AGE:         ○ NICU DAY # ____
○ HOME DAY # ____    WEIGHT:                  WEIGHT:                  ○ HOME DAY # ____

## Today We Got To

☐ PHONE CALL   ☐ SKIN TO SKIN   ☐ SING      ☐ PHONE CALL   ☐ SKIN TO SKIN   ☐ SING
☐ TOUCH        ☐ TAKE TEMP      ☐ BATH      ☐ TOUCH        ☐ TAKE TEMP      ☐ BATH
☐ DIAPER       ☐ FEEDING        ☐ MASSAGE   ☐ DIAPER       ☐ FEEDING        ☐ MASSAGE
☐ HOLD         ☐ READ           ☐ VISITORS  ☐ HOLD         ☐ READ           ☐ VISITORS

## Feedings

_____    _____
_____    _____
_____    _____
_____    _____
_____    _____
_____    _____
_____    _____
_____    _____

## Medical Stats

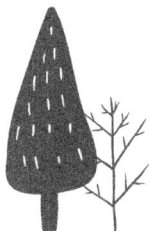
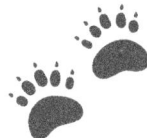

# Journaling

_____
_____
_____
_____
_____
_____
_____
_____
_____
_____
_____
_____
_____
_____
_____
_____
_____
_____

## QUESTIONS
TO ASK

Today I'm Grateful For...

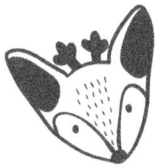
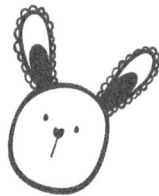

DATE:

_____       _____
NAME                   NAME

○ NICU DAY # ____    GESTATIONAL AGE:         GESTATIONAL AGE:       ○ NICU DAY # ____
○ HOME DAY # ____    WEIGHT:                  WEIGHT:            ○ HOME DAY # ____

## Today We Got To

| | | | | | |
|---|---|---|---|---|---|
| ☐ PHONE CALL | ☐ SKIN TO SKIN | ☐ SING | ☐ PHONE CALL | ☐ SKIN TO SKIN | ☐ SING |
| ☐ TOUCH | ☐ TAKE TEMP | ☐ BATH | ☐ TOUCH | ☐ TAKE TEMP | ☐ BATH |
| ☐ DIAPER | ☐ FEEDING | ☐ MASSAGE | ☐ DIAPER | ☐ FEEDING | ☐ MASSAGE |
| ☐ HOLD | ☐ READ | ☐ VISITORS | ☐ HOLD | ☐ READ | ☐ VISITORS |

## Feedings

_____    _____
_____    _____
_____    _____
_____    _____
_____    _____
_____    _____
_____    _____
_____    _____

## Medical Stats

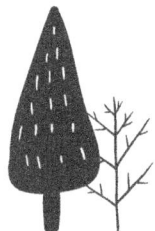
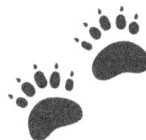

# Journaling

QUESTIONS
TO ASK

Today I'm Grateful For...

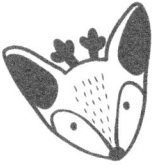
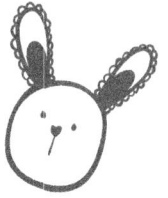

DATE:

_____          _____
NAME                                           NAME

○ NICU DAY # ____          GESTATIONAL AGE:          GESTATIONAL AGE:          ○ NICU DAY # ____
○ HOME DAY # ____          WEIGHT:                          WEIGHT:                          ○ HOME DAY # ____

## Today We Got To

☐ PHONE CALL   ☐ SKIN TO SKIN   ☐ SING          ☐ PHONE CALL   ☐ SKIN TO SKIN   ☐ SING
☐ TOUCH          ☐ TAKE TEMP       ☐ BATH         ☐ TOUCH          ☐ TAKE TEMP       ☐ BATH
☐ DIAPER         ☐ FEEDING          ☐ MASSAGE    ☐ DIAPER         ☐ FEEDING          ☐ MASSAGE
☐ HOLD            ☐ READ                ☐ VISITORS    ☐ HOLD            ☐ READ                ☐ VISITORS

## Feedings

_____          _____
_____          _____
_____          _____
_____          _____
_____          _____
_____          _____
_____          _____
_____          _____

## Medical Stats

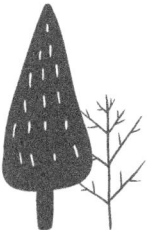
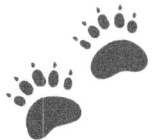

# Journaling

_____

_____

_____

_____

_____

_____

_____

_____

_____

_____

_____

_____

_____

QUESTIONS
TO ASK

_____

_____

_____

_____

Today I'm Grateful For...

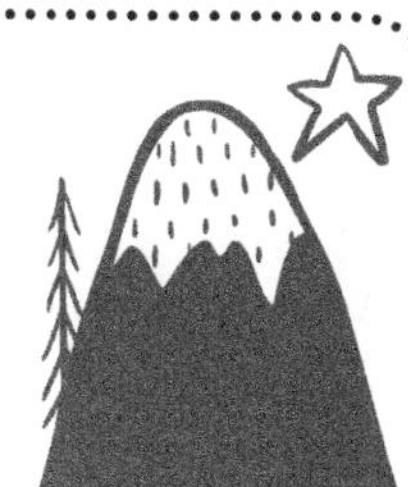

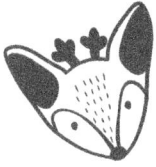
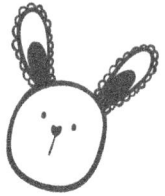

_____ NAME

NAME _____

○ NICU DAY # ____
○ HOME DAY # ____

GESTATIONAL AGE:

WEIGHT:

GESTATIONAL AGE:

WEIGHT:

○ NICU DAY # ____
○ HOME DAY # ____

## Today We Got To

☐ PHONE CALL  ☐ SKIN TO SKIN  ☐ SING
☐ TOUCH       ☐ TAKE TEMP     ☐ BATH
☐ DIAPER      ☐ FEEDING       ☐ MASSAGE
☐ HOLD        ☐ READ          ☐ VISITORS

☐ PHONE CALL  ☐ SKIN TO SKIN  ☐ SING
☐ TOUCH       ☐ TAKE TEMP     ☐ BATH
☐ DIAPER      ☐ FEEDING       ☐ MASSAGE
☐ HOLD        ☐ READ          ☐ VISITORS

## Feedings

## Medical Stats

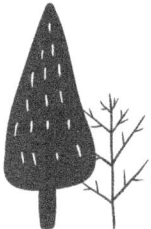
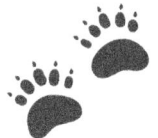

# Journaling

QUESTIONS
TO ASK

Today I'm Grateful For...

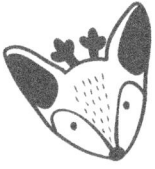
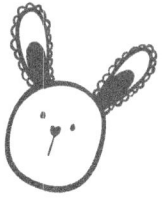

## DATE:

_____    _____
NAME    NAME

○ NICU DAY # ____
○ HOME DAY # ____

GESTATIONAL AGE:
WEIGHT:

GESTATIONAL AGE:
WEIGHT:

○ NICU DAY # ____
○ HOME DAY # ____

## Today We Got To

☐ PHONE CALL    ☐ SKIN TO SKIN    ☐ SING
☐ TOUCH    ☐ TAKE TEMP    ☐ BATH
☐ DIAPER    ☐ FEEDING    ☐ MASSAGE
☐ HOLD    ☐ READ    ☐ VISITORS

☐ PHONE CALL    ☐ SKIN TO SKIN    ☐ SING
☐ TOUCH    ☐ TAKE TEMP    ☐ BATH
☐ DIAPER    ☐ FEEDING    ☐ MASSAGE
☐ HOLD    ☐ READ    ☐ VISITORS

## Feedings

_____    _____
_____    _____
_____    _____
_____    _____
_____    _____
_____    _____
_____    _____
_____    _____

## Medical Stats

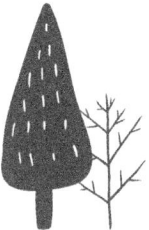
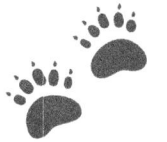

# Journaling

_____
_____
_____
_____
_____
_____
_____
_____
_____
_____
_____
_____
_____
_____
_____
_____
_____
_____

QUESTIONS
TO ASK

Today I'm Grateful For...

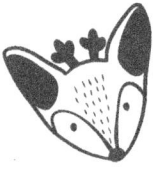
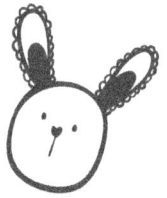

DATE:

_____
NAME

GESTATIONAL AGE:

WEIGHT:

○ NICU DAY # ____
○ HOME DAY # ____

_____
NAME

GESTATIONAL AGE:

WEIGHT:

○ NICU DAY # ____
○ HOME DAY # ____

## Today We Got To

☐ PHONE CALL    ☐ SKIN TO SKIN    ☐ SING
☐ TOUCH         ☐ TAKE TEMP       ☐ BATH
☐ DIAPER        ☐ FEEDING         ☐ MASSAGE
☐ HOLD          ☐ READ            ☐ VISITORS

☐ PHONE CALL    ☐ SKIN TO SKIN    ☐ SING
☐ TOUCH         ☐ TAKE TEMP       ☐ BATH
☐ DIAPER        ☐ FEEDING         ☐ MASSAGE
☐ HOLD          ☐ READ            ☐ VISITORS

## Feedings

_____    _____
_____    _____
_____    _____
_____    _____
_____    _____
_____    _____
_____    _____
_____    _____

## Medical Stats

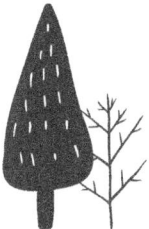
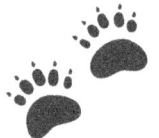

# Journaling

_____

_____

_____

_____

_____

_____

_____

_____

_____

_____

_____

_____

_____

_____

_____

_____

_____

_____

_____

## QUESTIONS
### TO ASK

## Today I'm Grateful For...

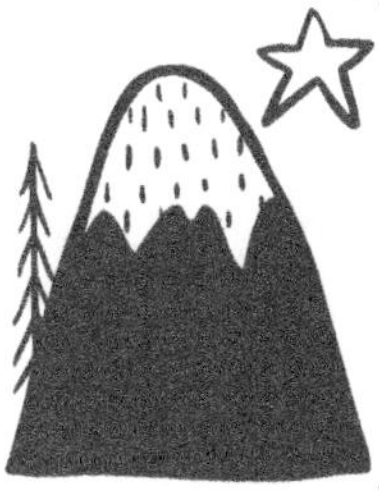

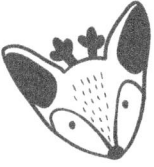
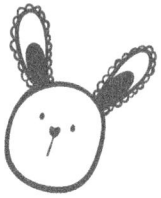

DATE:

_____      _____
NAME               NAME

○ NICU DAY # ____  GESTATIONAL AGE:      GESTATIONAL AGE:    ○ NICU DAY # ____
○ HOME DAY # ____  WEIGHT:          WEIGHT:          ○ HOME DAY # ____

## Today We Got To

☐ PHONE CALL    ☐ SKIN TO SKIN    ☐ SING        ☐ PHONE CALL    ☐ SKIN TO SKIN    ☐ SING
☐ TOUCH        ☐ TAKE TEMP     ☐ BATH        ☐ TOUCH        ☐ TAKE TEMP     ☐ BATH
☐ DIAPER       ☐ FEEDING       ☐ MASSAGE    ☐ DIAPER       ☐ FEEDING       ☐ MASSAGE
☐ HOLD         ☐ READ         ☐ VISITORS    ☐ HOLD         ☐ READ         ☐ VISITORS

## Feedings

_____      _____
_____      _____
_____      _____
_____      _____
_____      _____
_____      _____
_____      _____
_____      _____

## Medical Stats

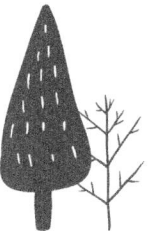
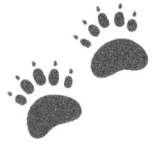

# Journaling

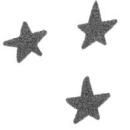

_____
_____
_____
_____
_____
_____
_____
_____
_____
_____
_____
_____
_____
_____
_____
_____
_____

## QUESTIONS
TO ASK

Today I'm Grateful For...

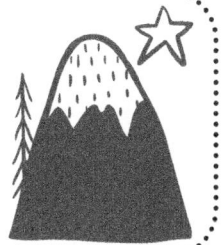

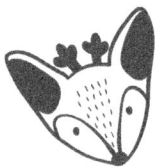

## DATE:

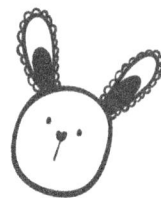

_____
NAME

_____
NAME

○ NICU DAY # ____
○ HOME DAY # ____

GESTATIONAL AGE:

WEIGHT:

GESTATIONAL AGE:

WEIGHT:

○ NICU DAY # ____
○ HOME DAY # ____

## Today We Got To

☐ PHONE CALL  ☐ SKIN TO SKIN  ☐ SING
☐ TOUCH        ☐ TAKE TEMP     ☐ BATH
☐ DIAPER       ☐ FEEDING       ☐ MASSAGE
☐ HOLD         ☐ READ          ☐ VISITORS

☐ PHONE CALL  ☐ SKIN TO SKIN  ☐ SING
☐ TOUCH        ☐ TAKE TEMP     ☐ BATH
☐ DIAPER       ☐ FEEDING       ☐ MASSAGE
☐ HOLD         ☐ READ          ☐ VISITORS

## Feedings

## Medical Stats

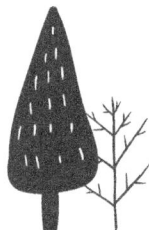

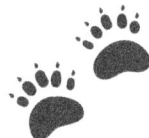

# Journaling

QUESTIONS
TO ASK

Today I'm Grateful For...

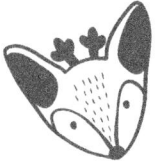
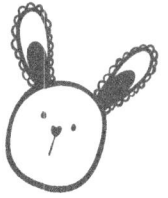

DATE:

_____  _____
NAME                        NAME

○ NICU DAY # ____     GESTATIONAL AGE: _____     GESTATIONAL AGE: _____     ○ NICU DAY # ____
○ HOME DAY # ____     WEIGHT: _____              WEIGHT: _____              ○ HOME DAY # ____

## Today We Got To

☐ PHONE CALL  ☐ SKIN TO SKIN  ☐ SING      ☐ PHONE CALL  ☐ SKIN TO SKIN  ☐ SING
☐ TOUCH       ☐ TAKE TEMP     ☐ BATH      ☐ TOUCH       ☐ TAKE TEMP     ☐ BATH
☐ DIAPER      ☐ FEEDING       ☐ MASSAGE   ☐ DIAPER      ☐ FEEDING       ☐ MASSAGE
☐ HOLD        ☐ READ          ☐ VISITORS  ☐ HOLD        ☐ READ          ☐ VISITORS

## Feedings

_____     _____
_____     _____
_____     _____
_____     _____
_____     _____
_____     _____
_____     _____
_____     _____

## Medical Stats

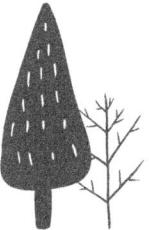
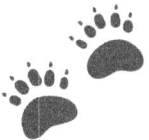

# Journaling

_____
_____
_____
_____
_____
_____
_____
_____
_____
_____
_____
_____
_____
_____
_____
_____
_____
_____

QUESTIONS
TO ASK

Today I'm Grateful For...

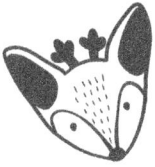
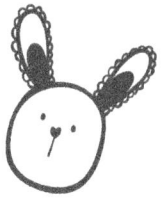

DATE:

_____ NAME _____    _____ NAME _____

○ NICU DAY # ____
○ HOME DAY # ____

GESTATIONAL AGE:

WEIGHT:

GESTATIONAL AGE:

WEIGHT:

○ NICU DAY # ____
○ HOME DAY # ____

## Today We Got To

☐ PHONE CALL    ☐ SKIN TO SKIN    ☐ SING
☐ TOUCH    ☐ TAKE TEMP    ☐ BATH
☐ DIAPER    ☐ FEEDING    ☐ MASSAGE
☐ HOLD    ☐ READ    ☐ VISITORS

☐ PHONE CALL    ☐ SKIN TO SKIN    ☐ SING
☐ TOUCH    ☐ TAKE TEMP    ☐ BATH
☐ DIAPER    ☐ FEEDING    ☐ MASSAGE
☐ HOLD    ☐ READ    ☐ VISITORS

## Feedings

_____    _____
_____    _____
_____    _____
_____    _____
_____    _____
_____    _____
_____    _____
_____    _____

## Medical Stats

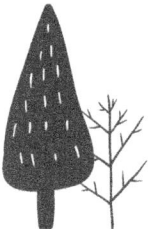
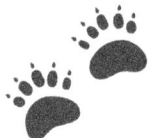

# Journaling

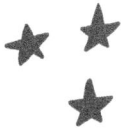

_____

_____

_____

_____

_____

_____

_____

_____

_____

_____

_____

_____

_____

## QUESTIONS
### TO ASK

_____

_____

_____

_____

_____

Today I'm Grateful For...

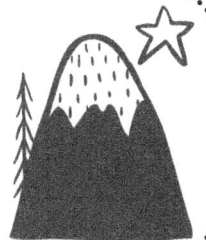

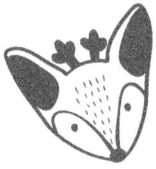

## DATE:

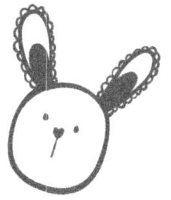

_____
NAME

_____
NAME

○ NICU DAY # ____
○ HOME DAY # ____

GESTATIONAL AGE:

WEIGHT:

GESTATIONAL AGE:

WEIGHT:

○ NICU DAY # ____
○ HOME DAY # ____

## Today We Got To

☐ PHONE CALL
☐ TOUCH
☐ DIAPER
☐ HOLD

☐ SKIN TO SKIN
☐ TAKE TEMP
☐ FEEDING
☐ READ

☐ SING
☐ BATH
☐ MASSAGE
☐ VISITORS

☐ PHONE CALL
☐ TOUCH
☐ DIAPER
☐ HOLD

☐ SKIN TO SKIN
☐ TAKE TEMP
☐ FEEDING
☐ READ

☐ SING
☐ BATH
☐ MASSAGE
☐ VISITORS

## Feedings

_____
_____
_____
_____
_____
_____
_____

_____
_____
_____
_____
_____
_____
_____

## Medical Stats

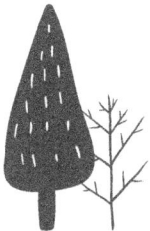

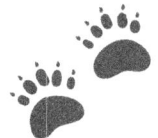

# Journaling

_____

_____

_____

_____

_____

_____

_____

_____

_____

_____

_____

_____

_____

_____

_____

_____

**QUESTIONS**
TO ASK

_____

_____

_____

_____

Today I'm Grateful For...

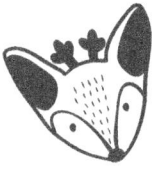
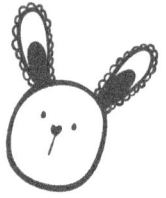

DATE:

_____    _____
NAME                          NAME

○ NICU DAY # ____    GESTATIONAL AGE:        GESTATIONAL AGE:        ○ NICU DAY # ____
○ HOME DAY # ____    WEIGHT:                 WEIGHT:                 ○ HOME DAY # ____

## Today We Got To

☐ PHONE CALL    ☐ SKIN TO SKIN    ☐ SING       ☐ PHONE CALL    ☐ SKIN TO SKIN    ☐ SING
☐ TOUCH         ☐ TAKE TEMP       ☐ BATH       ☐ TOUCH         ☐ TAKE TEMP       ☐ BATH
☐ DIAPER        ☐ FEEDING         ☐ MASSAGE    ☐ DIAPER        ☐ FEEDING         ☐ MASSAGE
☐ HOLD          ☐ READ            ☐ VISITORS   ☐ HOLD          ☐ READ            ☐ VISITORS

## Feedings

_____    _____
_____    _____
_____    _____
_____    _____
_____    _____
_____    _____
_____    _____
_____    _____

## Medical Stats

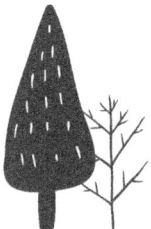
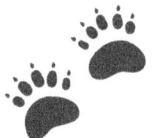

# Journaling

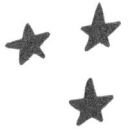

_____

_____

_____

_____

_____

_____

_____

_____

_____

_____

_____

_____

_____

## QUESTIONS
### TO ASK

Today I'm Grateful For...

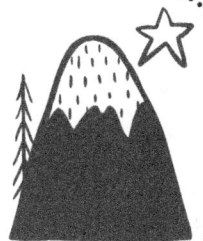

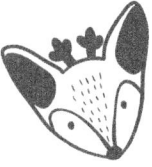
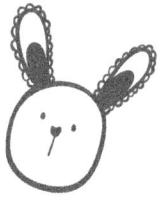

DATE:

_____ NAME
_____ NAME

○ NICU DAY # ___
○ HOME DAY # ___

GESTATIONAL AGE:

WEIGHT:

GESTATIONAL AGE:

WEIGHT:

○ NICU DAY # ___
○ HOME DAY # ___

## Today We Got To

□ PHONE CALL  □ SKIN TO SKIN  □ SING
□ TOUCH       □ TAKE TEMP     □ BATH
□ DIAPER      □ FEEDING       □ MASSAGE
□ HOLD        □ READ          □ VISITORS

□ PHONE CALL  □ SKIN TO SKIN  □ SING
□ TOUCH       □ TAKE TEMP     □ BATH
□ DIAPER      □ FEEDING       □ MASSAGE
□ HOLD        □ READ          □ VISITORS

## Feedings

_____          _____
_____          _____
_____          _____
_____          _____
_____          _____
_____          _____
_____          _____
_____          _____

## Medical Stats

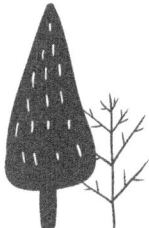
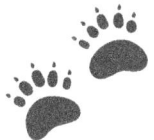

# Journaling

_____
_____
_____
_____
_____
_____
_____
_____
_____
_____
_____
_____
_____
_____
_____
_____
_____
_____

QUESTIONS
TO ASK

Today I'm Grateful For...

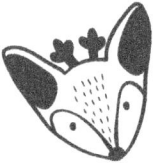

## DATE:

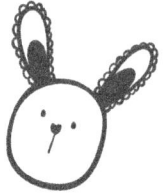

_____
NAME

_____
NAME

○ NICU DAY # ____
○ HOME DAY # ____

GESTATIONAL AGE:

WEIGHT:

GESTATIONAL AGE:

WEIGHT:

○ NICU DAY # ____
○ HOME DAY # ____

## Today We Got To

☐ PHONE CALL    ☐ SKIN TO SKIN    ☐ SING
☐ TOUCH    ☐ TAKE TEMP    ☐ BATH
☐ DIAPER    ☐ FEEDING    ☐ MASSAGE
☐ HOLD    ☐ READ    ☐ VISITORS

☐ PHONE CALL    ☐ SKIN TO SKIN    ☐ SING
☐ TOUCH    ☐ TAKE TEMP    ☐ BATH
☐ DIAPER    ☐ FEEDING    ☐ MASSAGE
☐ HOLD    ☐ READ    ☐ VISITORS

## Feedings

## Medical Stats

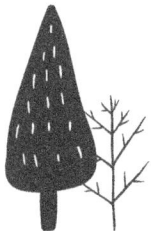

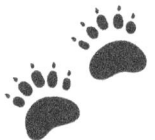

# Journaling

_____

_____

_____

_____

_____

_____

_____

_____

_____

_____

_____

_____

_____

_____

_____

_____

_____

_____

## QUESTIONS
### TO ASK

## Today I'm Grateful For...

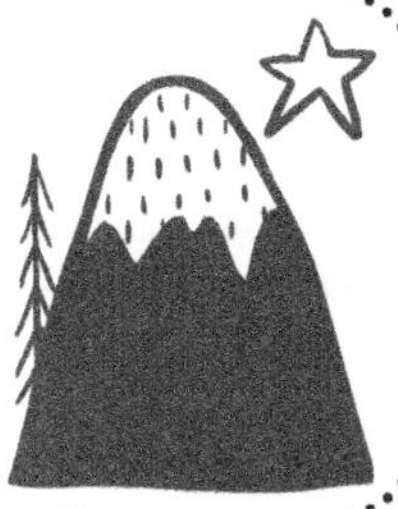

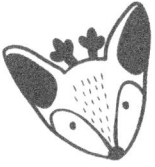
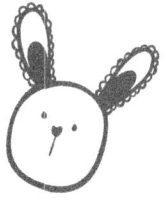

## DATE:

_____    _____
NAME    NAME

○ NICU DAY # ____     GESTATIONAL AGE:     GESTATIONAL AGE:     ○ NICU DAY # ____
○ HOME DAY # ____    WEIGHT:    WEIGHT:    ○ HOME DAY # ____

## Today We Got To

☐ PHONE CALL    ☐ SKIN TO SKIN    ☐ SING    ☐ PHONE CALL    ☐ SKIN TO SKIN    ☐ SING
☐ TOUCH    ☐ TAKE TEMP    ☐ BATH    ☐ TOUCH    ☐ TAKE TEMP    ☐ BATH
☐ DIAPER    ☐ FEEDING    ☐ MASSAGE    ☐ DIAPER    ☐ FEEDING    ☐ MASSAGE
☐ HOLD    ☐ READ    ☐ VISITORS    ☐ HOLD    ☐ READ    ☐ VISITORS

## Feedings

_____    _____
_____    _____
_____    _____
_____    _____
_____    _____
_____    _____
_____    _____
_____    _____

## Medical Stats

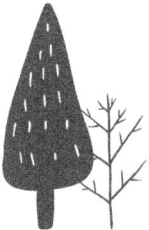
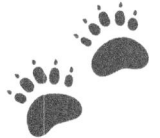

# Journaling

_____

_____

_____

_____

_____

_____

_____

_____

_____

_____

_____

_____

_____

_____

_____

## QUESTIONS
TO ASK

_____

_____

_____

_____

_____

Today I'm Grateful For...

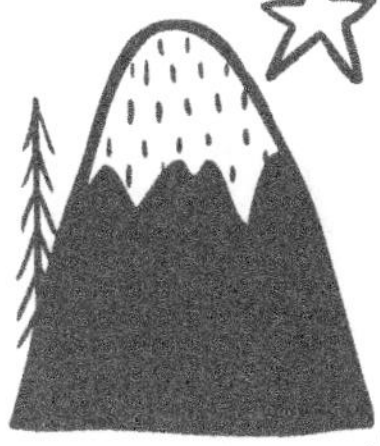

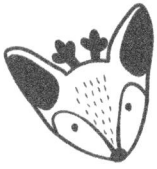
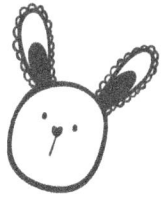

DATE:

_____
NAME

_____
NAME

○ NICU DAY # ____
○ HOME DAY # ____

GESTATIONAL AGE:

WEIGHT:

GESTATIONAL AGE:

WEIGHT:

○ NICU DAY # ____
○ HOME DAY # ____

## Today We Got To

☐ PHONE CALL     ☐ SKIN TO SKIN     ☐ SING
☐ TOUCH          ☐ TAKE TEMP        ☐ BATH
☐ DIAPER         ☐ FEEDING          ☐ MASSAGE
☐ HOLD           ☐ READ             ☐ VISITORS

☐ PHONE CALL     ☐ SKIN TO SKIN     ☐ SING
☐ TOUCH          ☐ TAKE TEMP        ☐ BATH
☐ DIAPER         ☐ FEEDING          ☐ MASSAGE
☐ HOLD           ☐ READ             ☐ VISITORS

## Feedings

_____     _____
_____     _____
_____     _____
_____     _____
_____     _____
_____     _____
_____     _____
_____     _____

## Medical Stats

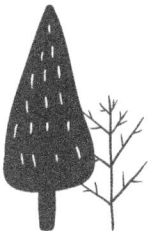
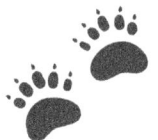

# Journaling

QUESTIONS
TO ASK

Today I'm Grateful For...

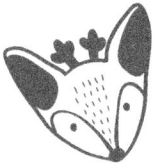
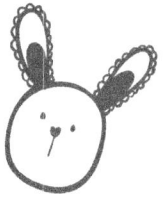

DATE:

_____          _____
NAME                                    NAME

○ NICU DAY # ____      GESTATIONAL AGE:        GESTATIONAL AGE:        ○ NICU DAY # ____
○ HOME DAY # ____     WEIGHT:                  WEIGHT:                 ○ HOME DAY # ____

## Today We Got To

☐ PHONE CALL    ☐ SKIN TO SKIN    ☐ SING      ☐ PHONE CALL    ☐ SKIN TO SKIN    ☐ SING
☐ TOUCH         ☐ TAKE TEMP       ☐ BATH      ☐ TOUCH         ☐ TAKE TEMP       ☐ BATH
☐ DIAPER        ☐ FEEDING         ☐ MASSAGE   ☐ DIAPER        ☐ FEEDING         ☐ MASSAGE
☐ HOLD          ☐ READ            ☐ VISITORS  ☐ HOLD          ☐ READ            ☐ VISITORS

## Feedings

_____          _____
_____          _____
_____          _____
_____          _____
_____          _____
_____          _____
_____          _____
_____          _____

## Medical Stats

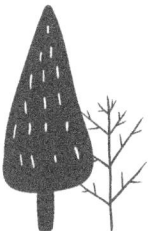
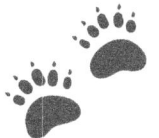

# Journaling

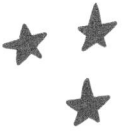

_____

_____

_____

_____

_____

_____

_____

_____

_____

_____

_____

_____

_____

_____

## QUESTIONS
### TO ASK

_____

_____

_____

_____

_____

Today I'm Grateful For...

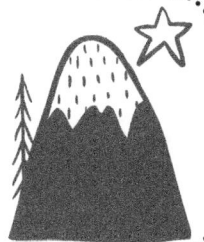

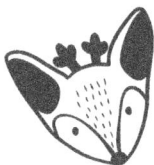
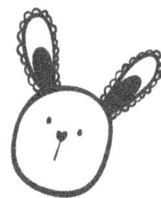

## DATE:

_____
NAME

_____
NAME

○ NICU DAY # _____
○ HOME DAY # _____

GESTATIONAL AGE:

WEIGHT:

GESTATIONAL AGE:

WEIGHT:

○ NICU DAY # _____
○ HOME DAY # _____

## Today We Got To

☐ PHONE CALL    ☐ SKIN TO SKIN    ☐ SING
☐ TOUCH    ☐ TAKE TEMP    ☐ BATH
☐ DIAPER    ☐ FEEDING    ☐ MASSAGE
☐ HOLD    ☐ READ    ☐ VISITORS

☐ PHONE CALL    ☐ SKIN TO SKIN    ☐ SING
☐ TOUCH    ☐ TAKE TEMP    ☐ BATH
☐ DIAPER    ☐ FEEDING    ☐ MASSAGE
☐ HOLD    ☐ READ    ☐ VISITORS

## Feedings

_____
_____
_____
_____
_____
_____
_____
_____
_____

_____
_____
_____
_____
_____
_____
_____
_____
_____

## Medical Stats

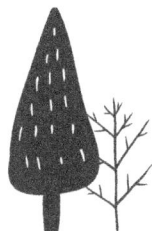
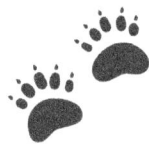

# Journaling

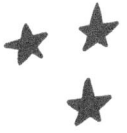

_____

_____

_____

_____

_____

_____

_____

_____

_____

_____

_____

_____

_____

## QUESTIONS
### TO ASK

_____

_____

_____

_____

_____

Today I'm Grateful For...

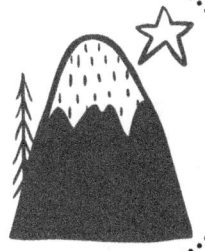

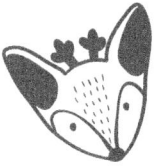
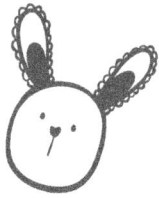

## DATE:

_____  |  _____
NAME  |  NAME

○ NICU DAY # ____     GESTATIONAL AGE: | GESTATIONAL AGE:     ○ NICU DAY # ____
○ HOME DAY # ____     WEIGHT: | WEIGHT:     ○ HOME DAY # ____

## Today We Got To

☐ PHONE CALL  ☐ SKIN TO SKIN  ☐ SING  |  ☐ PHONE CALL  ☐ SKIN TO SKIN  ☐ SING
☐ TOUCH       ☐ TAKE TEMP     ☐ BATH  |  ☐ TOUCH       ☐ TAKE TEMP     ☐ BATH
☐ DIAPER      ☐ FEEDING       ☐ MASSAGE  |  ☐ DIAPER      ☐ FEEDING       ☐ MASSAGE
☐ HOLD        ☐ READ          ☐ VISITORS  |  ☐ HOLD        ☐ READ          ☐ VISITORS

## Feedings

_____  |  _____
_____  |  _____
_____  |  _____
_____  |  _____
_____  |  _____
_____  |  _____
_____  |  _____
_____  |  _____

## Medical Stats

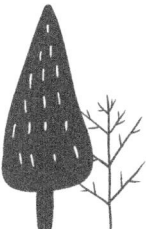
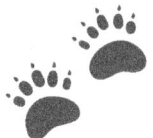

# Journaling

_____
_____
_____
_____
_____
_____
_____
_____
_____
_____
_____
_____
_____
_____
_____
_____
_____
_____

QUESTIONS
TO ASK

Today I'm Grateful For...

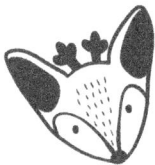
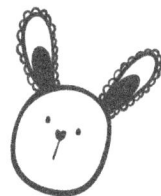

DATE:

_____
NAME

_____
NAME

○ NICU DAY # ____
○ HOME DAY # ____

GESTATIONAL AGE:

WEIGHT:

GESTATIONAL AGE:

WEIGHT:

○ NICU DAY # ____
○ HOME DAY # ____

## Today We Got To

☐ PHONE CALL      ☐ SKIN TO SKIN      ☐ SING          ☐ PHONE CALL      ☐ SKIN TO SKIN      ☐ SING
☐ TOUCH           ☐ TAKE TEMP         ☐ BATH          ☐ TOUCH           ☐ TAKE TEMP         ☐ BATH
☐ DIAPER          ☐ FEEDING           ☐ MASSAGE       ☐ DIAPER          ☐ FEEDING           ☐ MASSAGE
☐ HOLD            ☐ READ              ☐ VISITORS      ☐ HOLD            ☐ READ              ☐ VISITORS

## Feedings

_____        _____
_____        _____
_____        _____
_____        _____
_____        _____
_____        _____
_____        _____
_____        _____

## Medical Stats

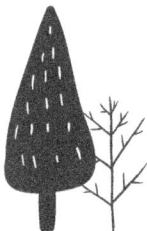
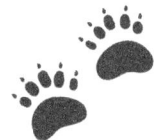

# Journaling

QUESTIONS
TO ASK

Today I'm Grateful For...

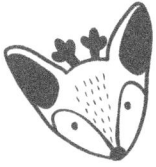
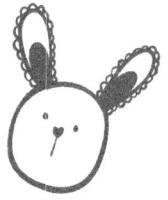

DATE:

_____ NAME

_____ NAME

○ NICU DAY # ____
○ HOME DAY # ____

GESTATIONAL AGE:

WEIGHT:

GESTATIONAL AGE:

WEIGHT:

○ NICU DAY # ____
○ HOME DAY # ____

## Today We Got To

☐ PHONE CALL  ☐ SKIN TO SKIN  ☐ SING
☐ TOUCH       ☐ TAKE TEMP     ☐ BATH
☐ DIAPER      ☐ FEEDING       ☐ MASSAGE
☐ HOLD        ☐ READ          ☐ VISITORS

☐ PHONE CALL  ☐ SKIN TO SKIN  ☐ SING
☐ TOUCH       ☐ TAKE TEMP     ☐ BATH
☐ DIAPER      ☐ FEEDING       ☐ MASSAGE
☐ HOLD        ☐ READ          ☐ VISITORS

## Feedings

_____
_____
_____
_____
_____
_____
_____
_____

_____
_____
_____
_____
_____
_____
_____
_____

## Medical Stats

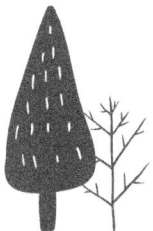
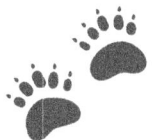

# Journaling

QUESTIONS
TO ASK

Today I'm Grateful For...

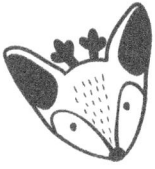
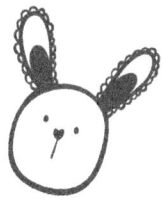

DATE:

_____
NAME

_____
NAME

○ NICU DAY # ____
○ HOME DAY # ____

GESTATIONAL AGE:

WEIGHT:

GESTATIONAL AGE:

WEIGHT:

○ NICU DAY # ____
○ HOME DAY # ____

## Today We Got To

☐ PHONE CALL
☐ TOUCH
☐ DIAPER
☐ HOLD

☐ SKIN TO SKIN
☐ TAKE TEMP
☐ FEEDING
☐ READ

☐ SING
☐ BATH
☐ MASSAGE
☐ VISITORS

☐ PHONE CALL
☐ TOUCH
☐ DIAPER
☐ HOLD

☐ SKIN TO SKIN
☐ TAKE TEMP
☐ FEEDING
☐ READ

☐ SING
☐ BATH
☐ MASSAGE
☐ VISITORS

## Feedings

_____
_____
_____
_____
_____
_____
_____
_____

_____
_____
_____
_____
_____
_____
_____
_____

## Medical Stats

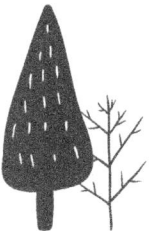
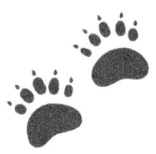

# Journaling

_____

_____

_____

_____

_____

_____

_____

_____

_____

_____

_____

_____

_____

_____

QUESTIONS
TO ASK

_____

_____

_____

_____

_____

Today I'm Grateful For...

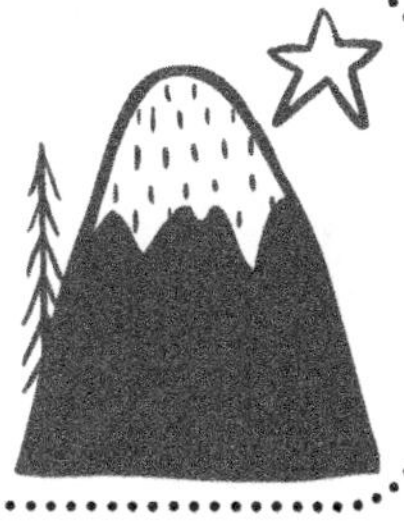

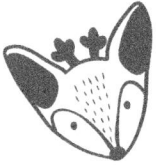
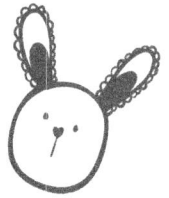

DATE:

_____ NAME _____        _____ NAME _____

○ NICU DAY # ____
○ HOME DAY # ____

GESTATIONAL AGE:

WEIGHT:

GESTATIONAL AGE:

WEIGHT:

○ NICU DAY # ____
○ HOME DAY # ____

## Today We Got To

☐ PHONE CALL  ☐ SKIN TO SKIN  ☐ SING
☐ TOUCH  ☐ TAKE TEMP  ☐ BATH
☐ DIAPER  ☐ FEEDING  ☐ MASSAGE
☐ HOLD  ☐ READ  ☐ VISITORS

☐ PHONE CALL  ☐ SKIN TO SKIN  ☐ SING
☐ TOUCH  ☐ TAKE TEMP  ☐ BATH
☐ DIAPER  ☐ FEEDING  ☐ MASSAGE
☐ HOLD  ☐ READ  ☐ VISITORS

## Feedings

_____
_____
_____
_____
_____
_____
_____
_____

_____
_____
_____
_____
_____
_____
_____
_____

## Medical Stats

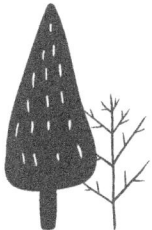
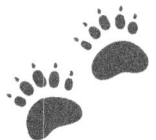

# Journaling

QUESTIONS
TO ASK

Today I'm Grateful For...

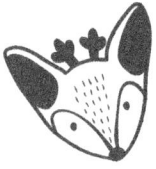
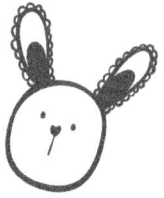

DATE:

_____  _____
NAME                                    NAME

○ NICU DAY # ____   GESTATIONAL AGE:     GESTATIONAL AGE:     ○ NICU DAY # ____
○ HOME DAY # ____   WEIGHT:              WEIGHT:              ○ HOME DAY # ____

## Today We Got To

☐ PHONE CALL   ☐ SKIN TO SKIN   ☐ SING       ☐ PHONE CALL   ☐ SKIN TO SKIN   ☐ SING
☐ TOUCH        ☐ TAKE TEMP      ☐ BATH       ☐ TOUCH        ☐ TAKE TEMP      ☐ BATH
☐ DIAPER       ☐ FEEDING        ☐ MASSAGE    ☐ DIAPER       ☐ FEEDING        ☐ MASSAGE
☐ HOLD         ☐ READ           ☐ VISITORS   ☐ HOLD         ☐ READ           ☐ VISITORS

## Feedings

_____   _____
_____   _____
_____   _____
_____   _____
_____   _____
_____   _____
_____   _____
_____   _____
_____   _____

## Medical Stats

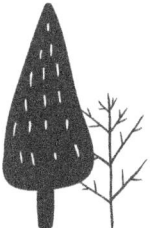
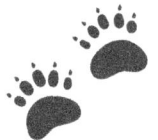

Journaling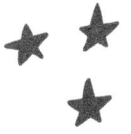

_____

_____

_____

_____

_____

_____

_____

_____

_____

_____

_____

_____

_____

_____

_____

QUESTIONS
TO ASK

_____

_____

_____

_____

_____

Today I'm Grateful For...

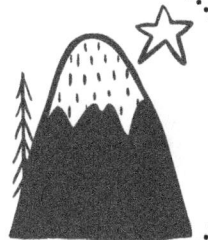

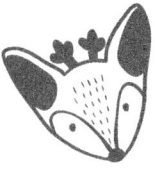
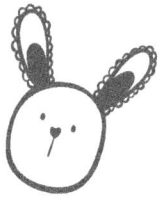

| DATE: |
|-------|

_____ NAME

_____ NAME

○ NICU DAY # ____
○ HOME DAY # ____

| GESTATIONAL AGE: |
| WEIGHT: |

| GESTATIONAL AGE: |
| WEIGHT: |

○ NICU DAY # ____
○ HOME DAY # ____

## Today We Got To

☐ PHONE CALL   ☐ SKIN TO SKIN   ☐ SING
☐ TOUCH        ☐ TAKE TEMP      ☐ BATH
☐ DIAPER       ☐ FEEDING        ☐ MASSAGE
☐ HOLD         ☐ READ           ☐ VISITORS

☐ PHONE CALL   ☐ SKIN TO SKIN   ☐ SING
☐ TOUCH        ☐ TAKE TEMP      ☐ BATH
☐ DIAPER       ☐ FEEDING        ☐ MASSAGE
☐ HOLD         ☐ READ           ☐ VISITORS

## Feedings

_____
_____
_____
_____
_____
_____
_____

_____
_____
_____
_____
_____
_____
_____

## Medical Stats

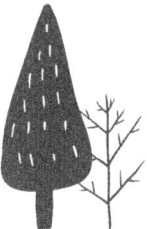
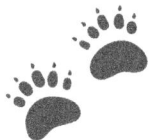

# Journaling

_____
_____
_____
_____
_____
_____
_____
_____
_____
_____
_____
_____
_____
_____
_____

QUESTIONS
TO ASK

_____
_____
_____
_____
_____

Today I'm Grateful For...

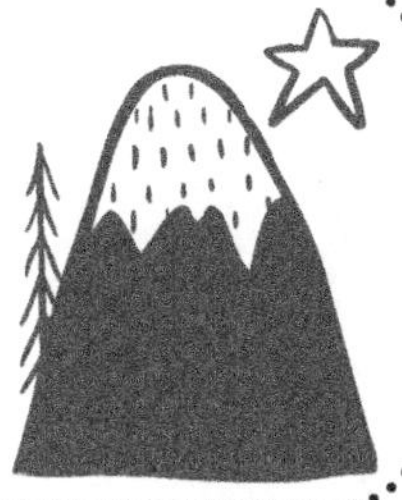

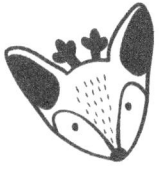
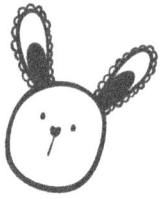

DATE:

_____ NAME

_____ NAME

○ NICU DAY # ____
○ HOME DAY # ____

GESTATIONAL AGE:

WEIGHT:

GESTATIONAL AGE:

WEIGHT:

○ NICU DAY # ____
○ HOME DAY # ____

## Today We Got To

☐ PHONE CALL    ☐ SKIN TO SKIN    ☐ SING
☐ TOUCH         ☐ TAKE TEMP       ☐ BATH
☐ DIAPER        ☐ FEEDING         ☐ MASSAGE
☐ HOLD          ☐ READ            ☐ VISITORS

☐ PHONE CALL    ☐ SKIN TO SKIN    ☐ SING
☐ TOUCH         ☐ TAKE TEMP       ☐ BATH
☐ DIAPER        ☐ FEEDING         ☐ MASSAGE
☐ HOLD          ☐ READ            ☐ VISITORS

## Feedings

## Medical Stats

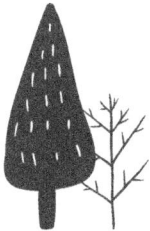
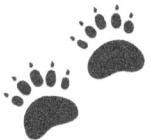

# Journaling

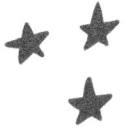

_____
_____
_____
_____
_____
_____
_____
_____
_____
_____
_____
_____
_____
_____
_____
_____
_____
_____

## QUESTIONS
TO ASK

Today I'm Grateful For...

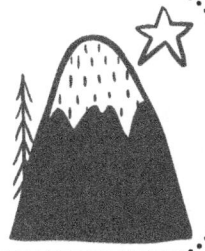

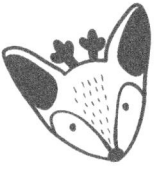
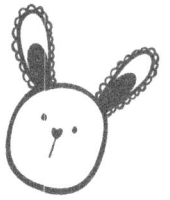

## DATE:

---

NAME                                        NAME

○ NICU DAY # ____    GESTATIONAL AGE:        GESTATIONAL AGE:        ○ NICU DAY # ____
○ HOME DAY # ____    WEIGHT:                 WEIGHT:                 ○ HOME DAY # ____

## Today We Got To

☐ PHONE CALL   ☐ SKIN TO SKIN   ☐ SING      ☐ PHONE CALL   ☐ SKIN TO SKIN   ☐ SING
☐ TOUCH        ☐ TAKE TEMP      ☐ BATH      ☐ TOUCH        ☐ TAKE TEMP      ☐ BATH
☐ DIAPER       ☐ FEEDING        ☐ MASSAGE   ☐ DIAPER       ☐ FEEDING        ☐ MASSAGE
☐ HOLD         ☐ READ           ☐ VISITORS  ☐ HOLD         ☐ READ           ☐ VISITORS

## Feedings

_____        _____
_____        _____
_____        _____
_____        _____
_____        _____
_____        _____
_____        _____
_____        _____

## Medical Stats

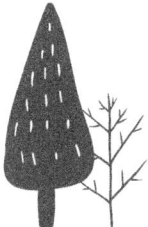
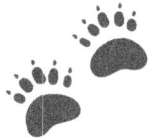

# Journaling

_____
_____
_____
_____
_____
_____
_____
_____
_____
_____
_____
_____
_____
_____
_____
_____
_____
_____
_____

QUESTIONS
TO ASK

Today I'm Grateful For...

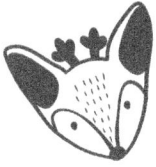
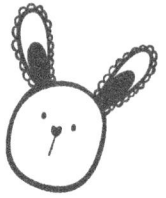

DATE:

_____
NAME

_____
NAME

○ NICU DAY # ____
○ HOME DAY # ____

GESTATIONAL AGE:

WEIGHT:

GESTATIONAL AGE:

WEIGHT:

○ NICU DAY # ____
○ HOME DAY # ____

## Today We Got To

- ☐ PHONE CALL
- ☐ TOUCH
- ☐ DIAPER
- ☐ HOLD

- ☐ SKIN TO SKIN
- ☐ TAKE TEMP
- ☐ FEEDING
- ☐ READ

- ☐ SING
- ☐ BATH
- ☐ MASSAGE
- ☐ VISITORS

- ☐ PHONE CALL
- ☐ TOUCH
- ☐ DIAPER
- ☐ HOLD

- ☐ SKIN TO SKIN
- ☐ TAKE TEMP
- ☐ FEEDING
- ☐ READ

- ☐ SING
- ☐ BATH
- ☐ MASSAGE
- ☐ VISITORS

## Feedings

## Medical Stats

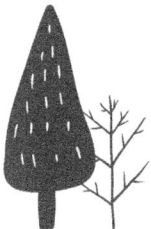
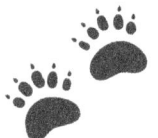

# Journaling

_____

_____

_____

_____

_____

_____

_____

_____

_____

_____

_____

_____

_____

## QUESTIONS
### TO ASK

_____

_____

_____

_____

_____

Today I'm Grateful For...

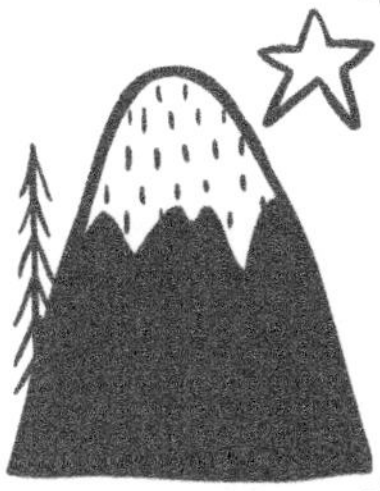

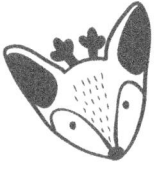
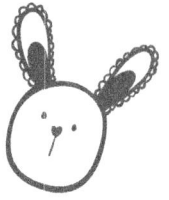

DATE:

_____          _____
NAME                                          NAME

○ NICU DAY # ___     GESTATIONAL AGE:          GESTATIONAL AGE:          ○ NICU DAY # ___
○ HOME DAY # ___     WEIGHT:                   WEIGHT:                   ○ HOME DAY # ___

## Today We Got To

☐ PHONE CALL   ☐ SKIN TO SKIN   ☐ SING      ☐ PHONE CALL   ☐ SKIN TO SKIN   ☐ SING
☐ TOUCH        ☐ TAKE TEMP      ☐ BATH      ☐ TOUCH        ☐ TAKE TEMP      ☐ BATH
☐ DIAPER       ☐ FEEDING        ☐ MASSAGE   ☐ DIAPER       ☐ FEEDING        ☐ MASSAGE
☐ HOLD         ☐ READ           ☐ VISITORS  ☐ HOLD         ☐ READ           ☐ VISITORS

## Feedings

_____          _____
_____          _____
_____          _____
_____          _____
_____          _____
_____          _____
_____          _____
_____          _____

## Medical Stats

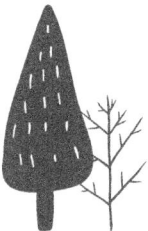
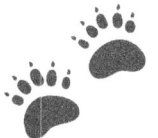

# Journaling

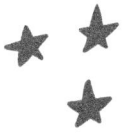

_____

_____

_____

_____

_____

_____

_____

_____

_____

_____

_____

_____

_____

## QUESTIONS
TO ASK

_____

_____

_____

_____

_____

Today I'm Grateful For...

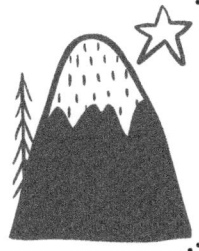

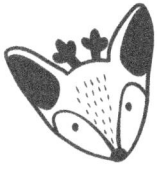
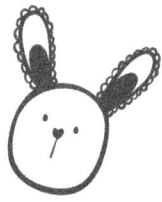

DATE:

_____ NAME

_____ NAME

○ NICU DAY # ____
○ HOME DAY # ____

GESTATIONAL AGE:

WEIGHT:

GESTATIONAL AGE:

WEIGHT:

○ NICU DAY # ____
○ HOME DAY # ____

## Today We Got To

☐ PHONE CALL   ☐ SKIN TO SKIN   ☐ SING
☐ TOUCH        ☐ TAKE TEMP      ☐ BATH
☐ DIAPER       ☐ FEEDING        ☐ MASSAGE
☐ HOLD         ☐ READ           ☐ VISITORS

☐ PHONE CALL   ☐ SKIN TO SKIN   ☐ SING
☐ TOUCH        ☐ TAKE TEMP      ☐ BATH
☐ DIAPER       ☐ FEEDING        ☐ MASSAGE
☐ HOLD         ☐ READ           ☐ VISITORS

## Feedings

_____
_____
_____
_____
_____
_____
_____
_____

_____
_____
_____
_____
_____
_____
_____
_____

## Medical Stats

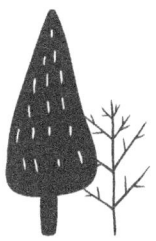
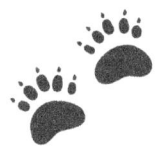

# Journaling

_____
_____
_____
_____
_____
_____
_____
_____
_____
_____
_____
_____
_____
_____
_____
_____
_____
_____
_____
_____
_____

## QUESTIONS
TO ASK

## Today I'm Grateful For...

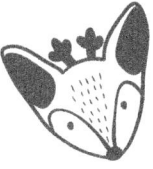
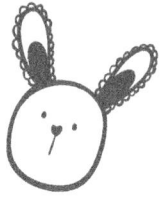

DATE:

_____
NAME

_____
NAME

○ NICU DAY # ____
○ HOME DAY # ____

GESTATIONAL AGE:

WEIGHT:

GESTATIONAL AGE:

WEIGHT:

○ NICU DAY # ____
○ HOME DAY # ____

## Today We Got To

☐ PHONE CALL  ☐ SKIN TO SKIN  ☐ SING
☐ TOUCH       ☐ TAKE TEMP     ☐ BATH
☐ DIAPER      ☐ FEEDING       ☐ MASSAGE
☐ HOLD        ☐ READ          ☐ VISITORS

☐ PHONE CALL  ☐ SKIN TO SKIN  ☐ SING
☐ TOUCH       ☐ TAKE TEMP     ☐ BATH
☐ DIAPER      ☐ FEEDING       ☐ MASSAGE
☐ HOLD        ☐ READ          ☐ VISITORS

## Feedings

_____
_____
_____
_____
_____
_____
_____
_____

_____
_____
_____
_____
_____
_____
_____
_____

## Medical Stats

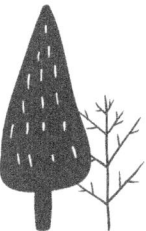
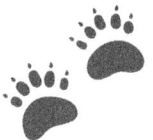

# Journaling

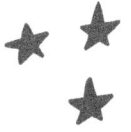

_____
_____
_____
_____
_____
_____
_____
_____
_____
_____
_____
_____
_____
_____
_____
_____
_____
_____
_____

## QUESTIONS
TO ASK

Today I'm Grateful For...

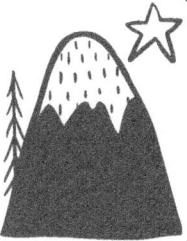

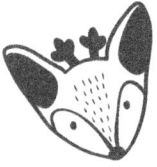
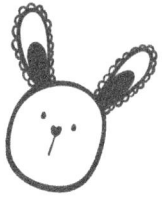

DATE:

_____ NAME

_____ NAME

○ NICU DAY # ____
○ HOME DAY # ____

GESTATIONAL AGE:

WEIGHT:

GESTATIONAL AGE:

WEIGHT:

○ NICU DAY # ____
○ HOME DAY # ____

## Today We Got To

☐ PHONE CALL ☐ SKIN TO SKIN ☐ SING
☐ TOUCH ☐ TAKE TEMP ☐ BATH
☐ DIAPER ☐ FEEDING ☐ MASSAGE
☐ HOLD ☐ READ ☐ VISITORS

☐ PHONE CALL ☐ SKIN TO SKIN ☐ SING
☐ TOUCH ☐ TAKE TEMP ☐ BATH
☐ DIAPER ☐ FEEDING ☐ MASSAGE
☐ HOLD ☐ READ ☐ VISITORS

## Feedings

_____
_____
_____
_____
_____
_____
_____
_____
_____

_____
_____
_____
_____
_____
_____
_____
_____
_____

## Medical Stats

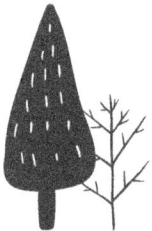
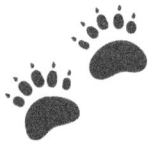

# Journaling

QUESTIONS
TO ASK

Today I'm Grateful For...

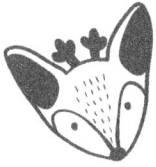
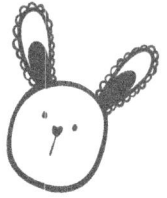

DATE:

_____ | _____
NAME | NAME

○ NICU DAY # ____
○ HOME DAY # ____

GESTATIONAL AGE:
WEIGHT:

GESTATIONAL AGE:
WEIGHT:

○ NICU DAY # ____
○ HOME DAY # ____

## Today We Got To

☐ PHONE CALL   ☐ SKIN TO SKIN   ☐ SING
☐ TOUCH        ☐ TAKE TEMP      ☐ BATH
☐ DIAPER       ☐ FEEDING        ☐ MASSAGE
☐ HOLD         ☐ READ           ☐ VISITORS

☐ PHONE CALL   ☐ SKIN TO SKIN   ☐ SING
☐ TOUCH        ☐ TAKE TEMP      ☐ BATH
☐ DIAPER       ☐ FEEDING        ☐ MASSAGE
☐ HOLD         ☐ READ           ☐ VISITORS

## Feedings

_____ | _____
_____ | _____
_____ | _____
_____ | _____
_____ | _____
_____ | _____
_____ | _____
_____ | _____

## Medical Stats

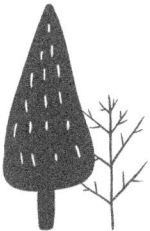
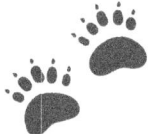

# Journaling

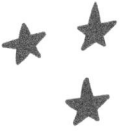

_____
_____
_____
_____
_____
_____
_____
_____
_____
_____
_____
_____
_____
_____
_____
_____
_____
_____
_____
_____

## QUESTIONS
TO ASK

Today I'm Grateful For...

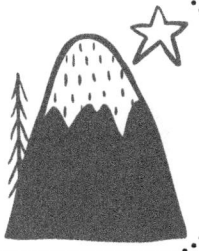

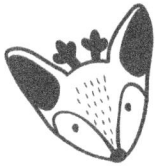
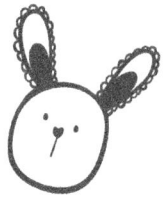

DATE:

_____
NAME

_____
NAME

○ NICU DAY # ____
○ HOME DAY # ____

GESTATIONAL AGE:

WEIGHT:

GESTATIONAL AGE:

WEIGHT:

○ NICU DAY # ____
○ HOME DAY # ____

## Today We Got To

☐ PHONE CALL    ☐ SKIN TO SKIN    ☐ SING
☐ TOUCH    ☐ TAKE TEMP    ☐ BATH
☐ DIAPER    ☐ FEEDING    ☐ MASSAGE
☐ HOLD    ☐ READ    ☐ VISITORS

☐ PHONE CALL    ☐ SKIN TO SKIN    ☐ SING
☐ TOUCH    ☐ TAKE TEMP    ☐ BATH
☐ DIAPER    ☐ FEEDING    ☐ MASSAGE
☐ HOLD    ☐ READ    ☐ VISITORS

## Feedings

_____
_____
_____
_____
_____
_____
_____

_____
_____
_____
_____
_____
_____
_____

## Medical Stats

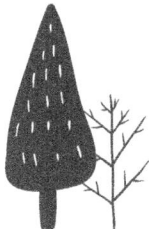
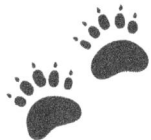

# Journaling

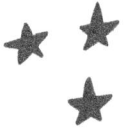

_____
_____
_____
_____
_____
_____
_____
_____
_____
_____
_____
_____
_____
_____
_____

## QUESTIONS
TO ASK

_____
_____
_____
_____
_____

Today I'm Grateful For...

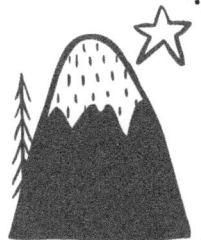

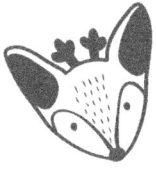
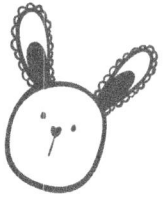

## DATE:

_____          _____
NAME                                            NAME

○ NICU DAY # ____          GESTATIONAL AGE:          GESTATIONAL AGE:          ○ NICU DAY # ____
○ HOME DAY # ____          WEIGHT:                          WEIGHT:                          ○ HOME DAY # ____

### Today We Got To

☐ PHONE CALL    ☐ SKIN TO SKIN    ☐ SING          ☐ PHONE CALL    ☐ SKIN TO SKIN    ☐ SING
☐ TOUCH              ☐ TAKE TEMP      ☐ BATH          ☐ TOUCH              ☐ TAKE TEMP      ☐ BATH
☐ DIAPER            ☐ FEEDING           ☐ MASSAGE    ☐ DIAPER            ☐ FEEDING           ☐ MASSAGE
☐ HOLD                ☐ READ                 ☐ VISITORS    ☐ HOLD                ☐ READ                 ☐ VISITORS

### Feedings

_____          _____
_____          _____
_____          _____
_____          _____
_____          _____
_____          _____
_____          _____
_____          _____

### Medical Stats

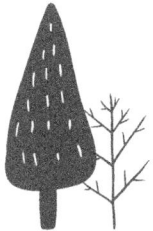
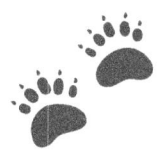

# Journaling

_____
_____
_____
_____
_____
_____
_____
_____
_____
_____
_____
_____
_____
_____
_____
_____
_____
_____
_____

QUESTIONS
TO ASK

Today I'm Grateful For...

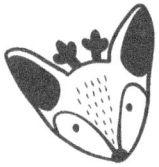
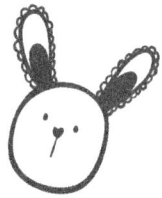

DATE:

_____                    _____
NAME                                        NAME

○ NICU DAY # ____     GESTATIONAL AGE:       GESTATIONAL AGE:        ○ NICU DAY # ____
○ HOME DAY # ____     WEIGHT:                WEIGHT:                 ○ HOME DAY # ____

## Today We Got To

☐ PHONE CALL   ☐ SKIN TO SKIN   ☐ SING       ☐ PHONE CALL   ☐ SKIN TO SKIN   ☐ SING
☐ TOUCH        ☐ TAKE TEMP      ☐ BATH       ☐ TOUCH        ☐ TAKE TEMP      ☐ BATH
☐ DIAPER       ☐ FEEDING        ☐ MASSAGE    ☐ DIAPER       ☐ FEEDING        ☐ MASSAGE
☐ HOLD         ☐ READ           ☐ VISITORS   ☐ HOLD         ☐ READ           ☐ VISITORS

## Feedings

_____                    _____
_____                    _____
_____                    _____
_____                    _____
_____                    _____
_____                    _____
_____                    _____
_____                    _____

## Medical Stats

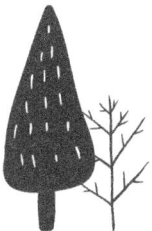
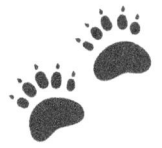

# Journaling

_____

_____

_____

_____

_____

_____

_____

_____

_____

_____

_____

_____

_____

_____

_____

## QUESTIONS
### TO ASK

_____

_____

_____

_____

_____

_____

Today I'm Grateful For...

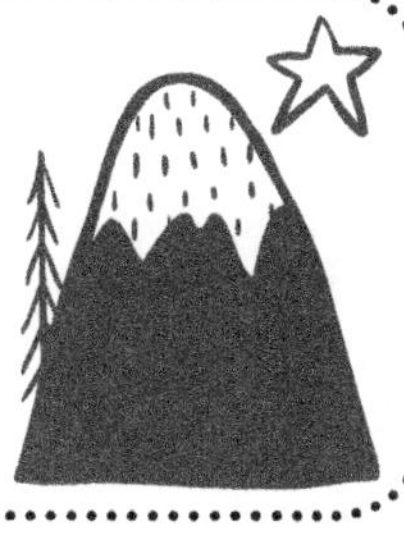

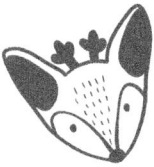
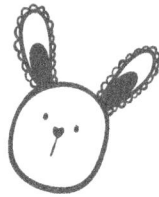

DATE:

_____          _____
NAME                                                      NAME

○ NICU DAY # ____          GESTATIONAL AGE:          GESTATIONAL AGE:          ○ NICU DAY # ____
○ HOME DAY # ____          WEIGHT:                          WEIGHT:                          ○ HOME DAY # ____

## Today We Got To

☐ PHONE CALL    ☐ SKIN TO SKIN    ☐ SING          ☐ PHONE CALL    ☐ SKIN TO SKIN    ☐ SING
☐ TOUCH               ☐ TAKE TEMP      ☐ BATH          ☐ TOUCH               ☐ TAKE TEMP      ☐ BATH
☐ DIAPER             ☐ FEEDING           ☐ MASSAGE    ☐ DIAPER             ☐ FEEDING           ☐ MASSAGE
☐ HOLD                 ☐ READ                 ☐ VISITORS     ☐ HOLD                 ☐ READ                 ☐ VISITORS

## Feedings

_____          _____
_____          _____
_____          _____
_____          _____
_____          _____
_____          _____
_____          _____
_____          _____
_____          _____

## Medical Stats

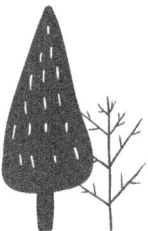
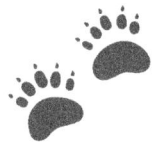

# Journaling

QUESTIONS
TO ASK

Today I'm Grateful For...

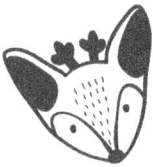
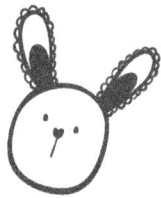

## DATE:

_____          _____
NAME                                            NAME

○ NICU DAY # ____     GESTATIONAL AGE:          GESTATIONAL AGE:     ○ NICU DAY # ____
○ HOME DAY # ____     WEIGHT:                    WEIGHT:              ○ HOME DAY # ____

## Today We Got To

☐ PHONE CALL  ☐ SKIN TO SKIN  ☐ SING      ☐ PHONE CALL  ☐ SKIN TO SKIN  ☐ SING
☐ TOUCH       ☐ TAKE TEMP     ☐ BATH      ☐ TOUCH       ☐ TAKE TEMP     ☐ BATH
☐ DIAPER      ☐ FEEDING       ☐ MASSAGE   ☐ DIAPER      ☐ FEEDING       ☐ MASSAGE
☐ HOLD        ☐ READ          ☐ VISITORS  ☐ HOLD        ☐ READ          ☐ VISITORS

## Feedings

_____          _____
_____          _____
_____          _____
_____          _____
_____          _____
_____          _____
_____          _____
_____          _____

## Medical Stats

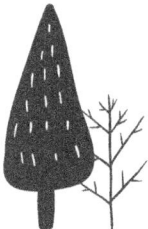
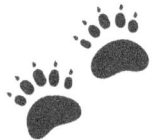

# Journaling

_____

_____

_____

_____

_____

_____

_____

_____

_____

_____

_____

_____

_____

_____

## QUESTIONS
### TO ASK

_____

_____

_____

_____

Today I'm Grateful For...

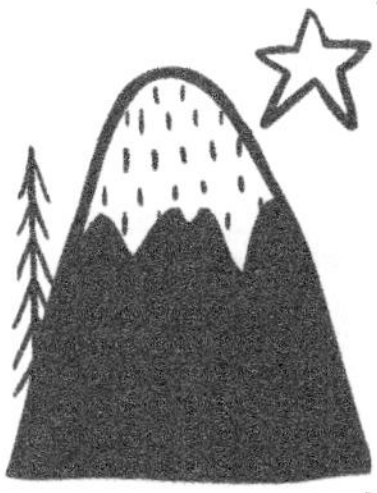

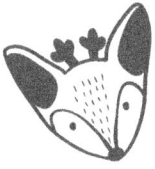
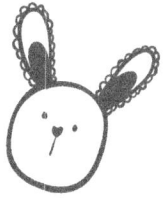

DATE:

_____  _____
NAME                              NAME

○ NICU DAY # ____    GESTATIONAL AGE:         GESTATIONAL AGE:         ○ NICU DAY # ____
○ HOME DAY # ____    WEIGHT:                  WEIGHT:                  ○ HOME DAY # ____

## Today We Got To

☐ PHONE CALL   ☐ SKIN TO SKIN   ☐ SING      ☐ PHONE CALL   ☐ SKIN TO SKIN   ☐ SING
☐ TOUCH        ☐ TAKE TEMP      ☐ BATH      ☐ TOUCH        ☐ TAKE TEMP      ☐ BATH
☐ DIAPER       ☐ FEEDING        ☐ MASSAGE   ☐ DIAPER       ☐ FEEDING        ☐ MASSAGE
☐ HOLD         ☐ READ           ☐ VISITORS  ☐ HOLD         ☐ READ           ☐ VISITORS

## Feedings

_____        _____
_____        _____
_____        _____
_____        _____
_____        _____
_____        _____
_____        _____
_____        _____

## Medical Stats

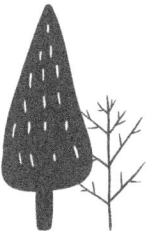
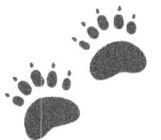

*Journaling*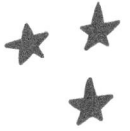

_____
_____
_____
_____
_____
_____
_____
_____
_____
_____
_____
_____
_____
_____

### QUESTIONS
TO ASK

_____
_____
_____
_____
_____

*Today I'm Grateful For...*

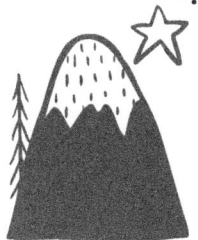

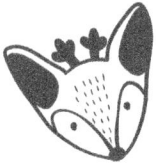
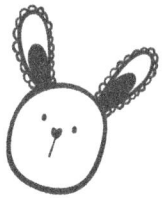

## DATE:

_____  _____
NAME                                    NAME

○ NICU DAY # ____
○ HOME DAY # ____

GESTATIONAL AGE:

WEIGHT:

GESTATIONAL AGE:

WEIGHT:

○ NICU DAY # ____
○ HOME DAY # ____

## Today We Got To

☐ PHONE CALL    ☐ SKIN TO SKIN    ☐ SING
☐ TOUCH             ☐ TAKE TEMP       ☐ BATH
☐ DIAPER            ☐ FEEDING            ☐ MASSAGE
☐ HOLD               ☐ READ                  ☐ VISITORS

☐ PHONE CALL    ☐ SKIN TO SKIN    ☐ SING
☐ TOUCH             ☐ TAKE TEMP       ☐ BATH
☐ DIAPER            ☐ FEEDING            ☐ MASSAGE
☐ HOLD               ☐ READ                  ☐ VISITORS

## Feedings

_____          _____
_____          _____
_____          _____
_____          _____
_____          _____
_____          _____
_____          _____
_____          _____

## Medical Stats

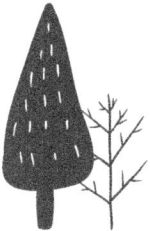
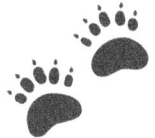

# Journaling

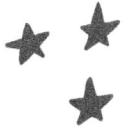

_____
_____
_____
_____
_____
_____
_____
_____
_____
_____
_____
_____
_____
_____
_____
_____
_____
_____
_____

### QUESTIONS
TO ASK

Today I'm Grateful For...

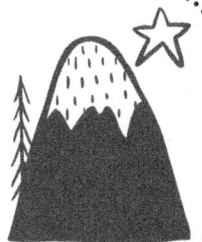

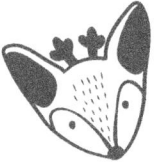
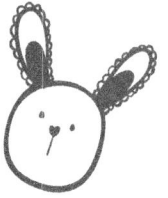

DATE:

_____ NAME

_____ NAME

○ NICU DAY # ___
○ HOME DAY # ___

GESTATIONAL AGE:

WEIGHT:

GESTATIONAL AGE:

WEIGHT:

○ NICU DAY # ___
○ HOME DAY # ___

## Today We Got To

☐ PHONE CALL   ☐ SKIN TO SKIN   ☐ SING        ☐ PHONE CALL   ☐ SKIN TO SKIN   ☐ SING
☐ TOUCH        ☐ TAKE TEMP       ☐ BATH        ☐ TOUCH        ☐ TAKE TEMP       ☐ BATH
☐ DIAPER       ☐ FEEDING         ☐ MASSAGE     ☐ DIAPER       ☐ FEEDING         ☐ MASSAGE
☐ HOLD         ☐ READ            ☐ VISITORS    ☐ HOLD         ☐ READ            ☐ VISITORS

## Feedings

_____    _____
_____    _____
_____    _____
_____    _____
_____    _____
_____    _____
_____    _____
_____    _____

## Medical Stats

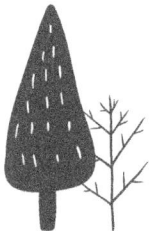
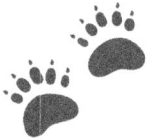

# Journaling

QUESTIONS
TO ASK

Today I'm Grateful For...

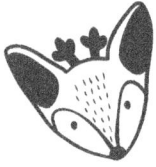
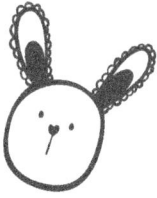

DATE:

_____
NAME

_____
NAME

○ NICU DAY # ____
○ HOME DAY # ____

GESTATIONAL AGE:

WEIGHT:

GESTATIONAL AGE:

WEIGHT:

○ NICU DAY # ____
○ HOME DAY # ____

## Today We Got To

□ PHONE CALL    □ SKIN TO SKIN    □ SING
□ TOUCH    □ TAKE TEMP    □ BATH
□ DIAPER    □ FEEDING    □ MASSAGE
□ HOLD    □ READ    □ VISITORS

□ PHONE CALL    □ SKIN TO SKIN    □ SING
□ TOUCH    □ TAKE TEMP    □ BATH
□ DIAPER    □ FEEDING    □ MASSAGE
□ HOLD    □ READ    □ VISITORS

## Feedings

_____
_____
_____
_____
_____
_____
_____
_____

_____
_____
_____
_____
_____
_____
_____
_____

## Medical Stats

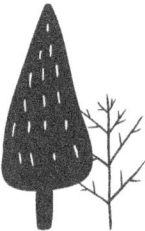
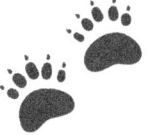

# Journaling

QUESTIONS
TO ASK

Today I'm Grateful For...

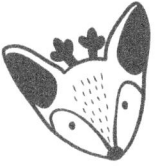
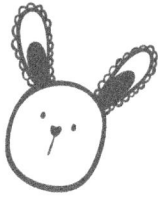

DATE:

_____
NAME

_____
NAME

○ NICU DAY # ____
○ HOME DAY # ____

GESTATIONAL AGE:

WEIGHT:

GESTATIONAL AGE:

WEIGHT:

○ NICU DAY # ____
○ HOME DAY # ____

## Today We Got To

☐ PHONE CALL  ☐ SKIN TO SKIN  ☐ SING
☐ TOUCH       ☐ TAKE TEMP     ☐ BATH
☐ DIAPER      ☐ FEEDING       ☐ MASSAGE
☐ HOLD        ☐ READ          ☐ VISITORS

☐ PHONE CALL  ☐ SKIN TO SKIN  ☐ SING
☐ TOUCH       ☐ TAKE TEMP     ☐ BATH
☐ DIAPER      ☐ FEEDING       ☐ MASSAGE
☐ HOLD        ☐ READ          ☐ VISITORS

## Feedings

_____
_____
_____
_____
_____
_____
_____
_____
_____

_____
_____
_____
_____
_____
_____
_____
_____

## Medical Stats

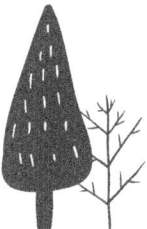
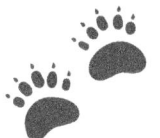

# Journaling

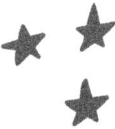

_____
_____
_____
_____
_____
_____
_____
_____
_____
_____
_____
_____
_____
_____
_____
_____
_____

## QUESTIONS
TO ASK

## Today I'm Grateful For...

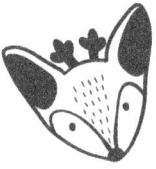
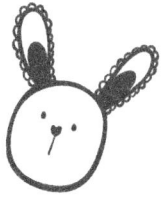

DATE:

_____  _____
NAME                                    NAME

○ NICU DAY # ____     GESTATIONAL AGE:          GESTATIONAL AGE:          ○ NICU DAY # ____
○ HOME DAY # ____     WEIGHT:                   WEIGHT:                   ○ HOME DAY # ____

## Today We Got To

☐ PHONE CALL   ☐ SKIN TO SKIN   ☐ SING       ☐ PHONE CALL   ☐ SKIN TO SKIN   ☐ SING
☐ TOUCH        ☐ TAKE TEMP      ☐ BATH       ☐ TOUCH        ☐ TAKE TEMP      ☐ BATH
☐ DIAPER       ☐ FEEDING        ☐ MASSAGE    ☐ DIAPER       ☐ FEEDING        ☐ MASSAGE
☐ HOLD         ☐ READ           ☐ VISITORS   ☐ HOLD         ☐ READ           ☐ VISITORS

## Feedings

_____        _____
_____        _____
_____        _____
_____        _____
_____        _____
_____        _____
_____        _____
_____        _____

## Medical Stats

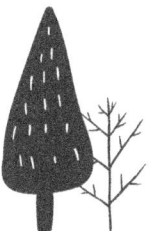
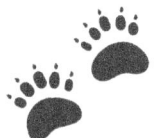

# Journaling

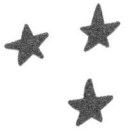

_____
_____
_____
_____
_____
_____
_____
_____
_____
_____
_____
_____
_____
_____
_____
_____

## QUESTIONS
TO ASK

_____
_____
_____
_____

Today I'm Grateful For...

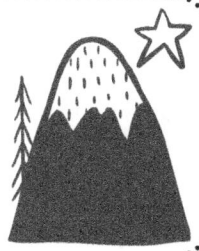

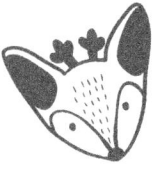
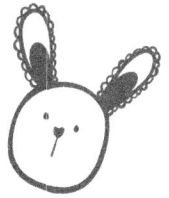

DATE:

_____                    _____
NAME                                              NAME

○ NICU DAY # ____          GESTATIONAL AGE:        GESTATIONAL AGE:          ○ NICU DAY # ____
○ HOME DAY # ____          WEIGHT:                 WEIGHT:                   ○ HOME DAY # ____

## Today We Got To

☐ PHONE CALL    ☐ SKIN TO SKIN    ☐ SING       ☐ PHONE CALL    ☐ SKIN TO SKIN    ☐ SING
☐ TOUCH         ☐ TAKE TEMP       ☐ BATH       ☐ TOUCH         ☐ TAKE TEMP       ☐ BATH
☐ DIAPER        ☐ FEEDING         ☐ MASSAGE    ☐ DIAPER        ☐ FEEDING         ☐ MASSAGE
☐ HOLD          ☐ READ            ☐ VISITORS   ☐ HOLD          ☐ READ            ☐ VISITORS

## Feedings

_____                    _____
_____                    _____
_____                    _____
_____                    _____
_____                    _____
_____                    _____
_____                    _____
_____                    _____

## Medical Stats

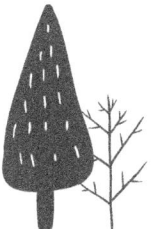
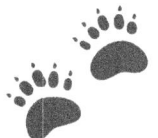

# Journaling

QUESTIONS
TO ASK

Today I'm Grateful For...

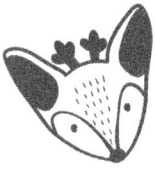
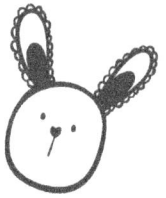

DATE:

_____ NAME

_____ NAME

○ NICU DAY # ____
○ HOME DAY # ____

GESTATIONAL AGE:

WEIGHT:

GESTATIONAL AGE:

WEIGHT:

○ NICU DAY # ____
○ HOME DAY # ____

## Today We Got To

☐ PHONE CALL   ☐ SKIN TO SKIN   ☐ SING
☐ TOUCH         ☐ TAKE TEMP      ☐ BATH
☐ DIAPER        ☐ FEEDING        ☐ MASSAGE
☐ HOLD          ☐ READ           ☐ VISITORS

☐ PHONE CALL   ☐ SKIN TO SKIN   ☐ SING
☐ TOUCH         ☐ TAKE TEMP      ☐ BATH
☐ DIAPER        ☐ FEEDING        ☐ MASSAGE
☐ HOLD          ☐ READ           ☐ VISITORS

## Feedings

_____
_____
_____
_____
_____
_____
_____
_____

_____
_____
_____
_____
_____
_____
_____
_____

## Medical Stats

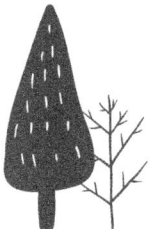
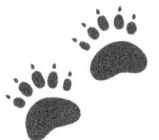

# Journaling

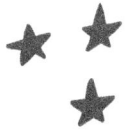

---
---
---
---
---
---
---
---
---
---
---
---
---
---
---
---
---
---
---
---
---
---

## QUESTIONS
### TO ASK

Today I'm Grateful For...

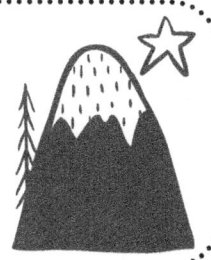

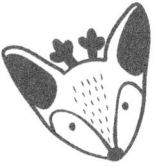
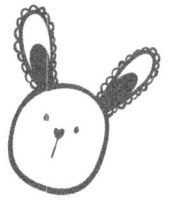

DATE:

_____ NAME

NAME _____

○ NICU DAY # ____
○ HOME DAY # ____

GESTATIONAL AGE:

WEIGHT:

GESTATIONAL AGE:

WEIGHT:

○ NICU DAY # ____
○ HOME DAY # ____

## Today We Got To

☐ PHONE CALL ☐ SKIN TO SKIN ☐ SING
☐ TOUCH ☐ TAKE TEMP ☐ BATH
☐ DIAPER ☐ FEEDING ☐ MASSAGE
☐ HOLD ☐ READ ☐ VISITORS

☐ PHONE CALL ☐ SKIN TO SKIN ☐ SING
☐ TOUCH ☐ TAKE TEMP ☐ BATH
☐ DIAPER ☐ FEEDING ☐ MASSAGE
☐ HOLD ☐ READ ☐ VISITORS

## Feedings

_____
_____
_____
_____
_____
_____
_____
_____

_____
_____
_____
_____
_____
_____
_____
_____

## Medical Stats

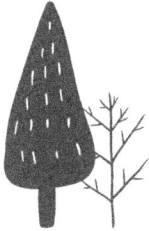
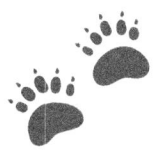

# Journaling

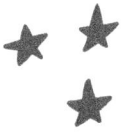

_____

_____

_____

_____

_____

_____

_____

_____

_____

_____

_____

_____

_____

_____

_____

_____

_____

_____

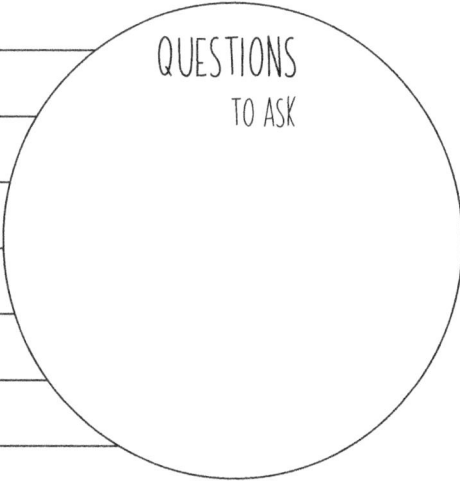

QUESTIONS
TO ASK

Today I'm Grateful For...

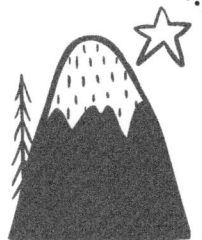

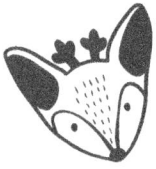
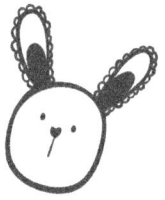

DATE:

_____          _____
NAME                                      NAME

○ NICU DAY # ___     GESTATIONAL AGE:          GESTATIONAL AGE:     ○ NICU DAY # ___
○ HOME DAY # ___     WEIGHT:                    WEIGHT:              ○ HOME DAY # ___

## Today We Got To

☐ PHONE CALL   ☐ SKIN TO SKIN   ☐ SING       ☐ PHONE CALL   ☐ SKIN TO SKIN   ☐ SING
☐ TOUCH        ☐ TAKE TEMP      ☐ BATH       ☐ TOUCH        ☐ TAKE TEMP      ☐ BATH
☐ DIAPER       ☐ FEEDING        ☐ MASSAGE    ☐ DIAPER       ☐ FEEDING        ☐ MASSAGE
☐ HOLD         ☐ READ           ☐ VISITORS   ☐ HOLD         ☐ READ           ☐ VISITORS

## Feedings

_____          _____
_____          _____
_____          _____
_____          _____
_____          _____
_____          _____
_____          _____
_____          _____

## Medical Stats

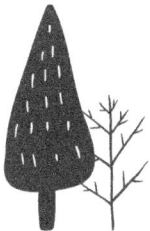
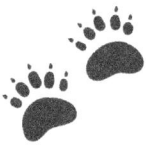

# Journaling

QUESTIONS
TO ASK

Today I'm Grateful For...

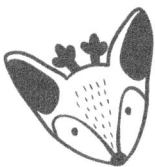
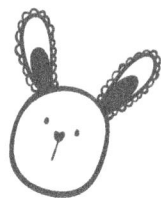

DATE:

_____
NAME

_____
NAME

○ NICU DAY # ____
○ HOME DAY # ____

GESTATIONAL AGE:

WEIGHT:

GESTATIONAL AGE:

WEIGHT:

○ NICU DAY # ____
○ HOME DAY # ____

## Today We Got To

☐ PHONE CALL  ☐ SKIN TO SKIN  ☐ SING
☐ TOUCH       ☐ TAKE TEMP     ☐ BATH
☐ DIAPER      ☐ FEEDING       ☐ MASSAGE
☐ HOLD        ☐ READ          ☐ VISITORS

☐ PHONE CALL  ☐ SKIN TO SKIN  ☐ SING
☐ TOUCH       ☐ TAKE TEMP     ☐ BATH
☐ DIAPER      ☐ FEEDING       ☐ MASSAGE
☐ HOLD        ☐ READ          ☐ VISITORS

## Feedings

_____
_____
_____
_____
_____
_____
_____

_____
_____
_____
_____
_____
_____
_____

## Medical Stats

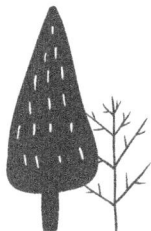
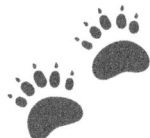

# Journaling

_____
_____
_____
_____
_____
_____
_____
_____
_____
_____
_____
_____
_____
_____
_____

## QUESTIONS
### TO ASK

Today I'm Grateful For...

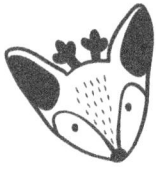
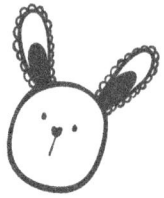

| DATE: |
| --- |

_____
NAME

_____
NAME

○ NICU DAY # ____
○ HOME DAY # ____

| GESTATIONAL AGE: | GESTATIONAL AGE: |
| --- | --- |
| WEIGHT: | WEIGHT: |

○ NICU DAY # ____
○ HOME DAY # ____

## Today We Got To

☐ PHONE CALL    ☐ SKIN TO SKIN    ☐ SING
☐ TOUCH    ☐ TAKE TEMP    ☐ BATH
☐ DIAPER    ☐ FEEDING    ☐ MASSAGE
☐ HOLD    ☐ READ    ☐ VISITORS

☐ PHONE CALL    ☐ SKIN TO SKIN    ☐ SING
☐ TOUCH    ☐ TAKE TEMP    ☐ BATH
☐ DIAPER    ☐ FEEDING    ☐ MASSAGE
☐ HOLD    ☐ READ    ☐ VISITORS

## Feedings

_____
_____
_____
_____
_____
_____
_____
_____
_____

## Medical Stats

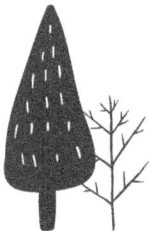
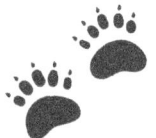

# Journaling

_____

_____

_____

_____

_____

_____

_____

_____

_____

_____

_____

_____

_____

_____

_____

_____

## QUESTIONS
TO ASK

## Today I'm Grateful For...

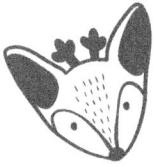
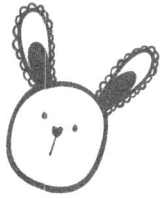

**DATE:**

_____          _____
NAME                                    NAME

○ NICU DAY # ____          GESTATIONAL AGE:          GESTATIONAL AGE:          ○ NICU DAY # ____
○ HOME DAY # ____          WEIGHT:                       WEIGHT:                       ○ HOME DAY # ____

## Today We Got To

☐ PHONE CALL     ☐ SKIN TO SKIN     ☐ SING          ☐ PHONE CALL     ☐ SKIN TO SKIN     ☐ SING
☐ TOUCH            ☐ TAKE TEMP        ☐ BATH          ☐ TOUCH            ☐ TAKE TEMP        ☐ BATH
☐ DIAPER           ☐ FEEDING           ☐ MASSAGE     ☐ DIAPER           ☐ FEEDING           ☐ MASSAGE
☐ HOLD              ☐ READ               ☐ VISITORS     ☐ HOLD              ☐ READ               ☐ VISITORS

## Feedings

_____          _____
_____          _____
_____          _____
_____          _____
_____          _____
_____          _____
_____          _____
_____          _____

## Medical Stats

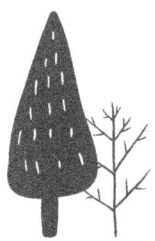
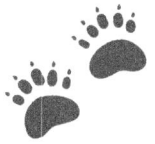

# Journaling

QUESTIONS
TO ASK

Today I'm Grateful For...

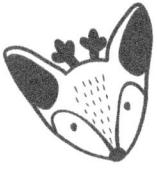
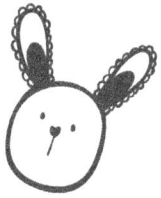

| DATE: |
|---|

_____  
NAME

_____  
NAME

○ NICU DAY # ____  
○ HOME DAY # ____

| GESTATIONAL AGE: |
| WEIGHT: |

| GESTATIONAL AGE: |
| WEIGHT: |

○ NICU DAY # ____  
○ HOME DAY # ____

## Today We Got To

☐ PHONE CALL  ☐ SKIN TO SKIN  ☐ SING  
☐ TOUCH  ☐ TAKE TEMP  ☐ BATH  
☐ DIAPER  ☐ FEEDING  ☐ MASSAGE  
☐ HOLD  ☐ READ  ☐ VISITORS  

☐ PHONE CALL  ☐ SKIN TO SKIN  ☐ SING  
☐ TOUCH  ☐ TAKE TEMP  ☐ BATH  
☐ DIAPER  ☐ FEEDING  ☐ MASSAGE  
☐ HOLD  ☐ READ  ☐ VISITORS  

## Feedings

_____  
_____  
_____  
_____  
_____  
_____  
_____  
_____  

_____  
_____  
_____  
_____  
_____  
_____  
_____  
_____  

## Medical Stats

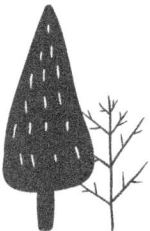
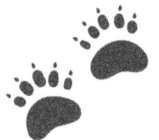

# Journaling

_____

_____

_____

_____

_____

_____

_____

_____

_____

_____

_____

_____

_____

## QUESTIONS
TO ASK

_____

_____

_____

_____

Today I'm Grateful For...

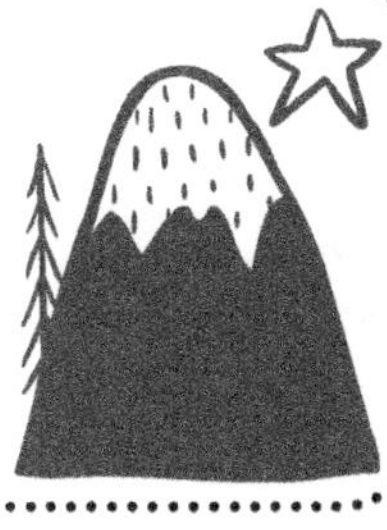

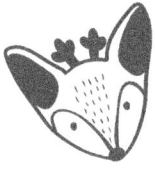
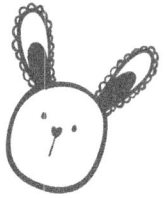

DATE:

_____ NAME

_____ NAME

○ NICU DAY # ___
○ HOME DAY # ___

GESTATIONAL AGE:

WEIGHT:

GESTATIONAL AGE:

WEIGHT:

○ NICU DAY # ___
○ HOME DAY # ___

## Today We Got To

- ☐ PHONE CALL
- ☐ TOUCH
- ☐ DIAPER
- ☐ HOLD

- ☐ SKIN TO SKIN
- ☐ TAKE TEMP
- ☐ FEEDING
- ☐ READ

- ☐ SING
- ☐ BATH
- ☐ MASSAGE
- ☐ VISITORS

- ☐ PHONE CALL
- ☐ TOUCH
- ☐ DIAPER
- ☐ HOLD

- ☐ SKIN TO SKIN
- ☐ TAKE TEMP
- ☐ FEEDING
- ☐ READ

- ☐ SING
- ☐ BATH
- ☐ MASSAGE
- ☐ VISITORS

## Feedings

## Medical Stats

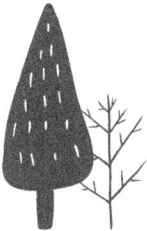
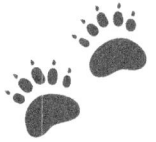

# Journaling

_____
_____
_____
_____
_____
_____
_____
_____
_____
_____
_____
_____
_____
_____
_____
_____
_____
_____

QUESTIONS
TO ASK

Today I'm Grateful For...

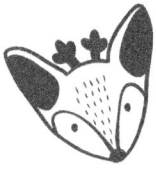
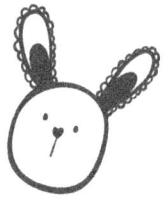

DATE:

_____ NAME       _____ NAME

○ NICU DAY # ____
○ HOME DAY # ____

GESTATIONAL AGE:

WEIGHT:

GESTATIONAL AGE:

WEIGHT:

○ NICU DAY # ____
○ HOME DAY # ____

## Today We Got To

☐ PHONE CALL    ☐ SKIN TO SKIN    ☐ SING
☐ TOUCH    ☐ TAKE TEMP    ☐ BATH
☐ DIAPER    ☐ FEEDING    ☐ MASSAGE
☐ HOLD    ☐ READ    ☐ VISITORS

☐ PHONE CALL    ☐ SKIN TO SKIN    ☐ SING
☐ TOUCH    ☐ TAKE TEMP    ☐ BATH
☐ DIAPER    ☐ FEEDING    ☐ MASSAGE
☐ HOLD    ☐ READ    ☐ VISITORS

## Feedings

## Medical Stats

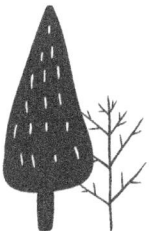
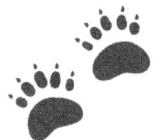

# Journaling

_____
_____
_____
_____
_____
_____
_____
_____
_____
_____
_____
_____
_____
_____
_____
_____

## QUESTIONS
TO ASK

## Today I'm Grateful For...

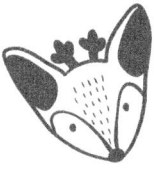
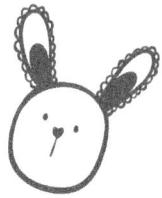

DATE:

NAME

NAME

○ NICU DAY # ____
○ HOME DAY # ____

GESTATIONAL AGE:

WEIGHT:

GESTATIONAL AGE:

WEIGHT:

○ NICU DAY # ____
○ HOME DAY # ____

## Today We Got To

☐ PHONE CALL  ☐ SKIN TO SKIN  ☐ SING
☐ TOUCH        ☐ TAKE TEMP     ☐ BATH
☐ DIAPER       ☐ FEEDING       ☐ MASSAGE
☐ HOLD         ☐ READ          ☐ VISITORS

☐ PHONE CALL  ☐ SKIN TO SKIN  ☐ SING
☐ TOUCH        ☐ TAKE TEMP     ☐ BATH
☐ DIAPER       ☐ FEEDING       ☐ MASSAGE
☐ HOLD         ☐ READ          ☐ VISITORS

## Feedings

_____          _____
_____          _____
_____          _____
_____          _____
_____          _____
_____          _____
_____          _____
_____          _____

## Medical Stats

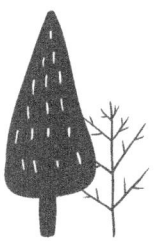
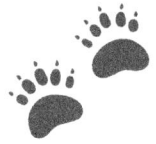

# Journaling

_____

_____

_____

_____

_____

_____

_____

_____

_____

_____

_____

_____

_____

## QUESTIONS
### TO ASK

_____

_____

_____

_____

_____

Today I'm Grateful For...

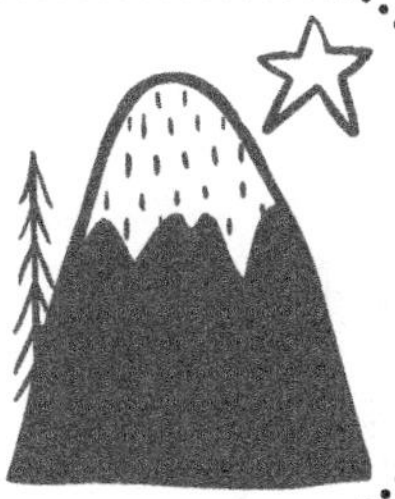

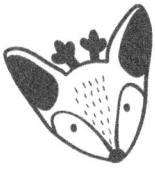
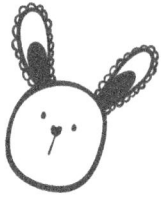

DATE:

_____
NAME

GESTATIONAL AGE:

WEIGHT:

○ NICU DAY # ____
○ HOME DAY # ____

_____
NAME

GESTATIONAL AGE:

WEIGHT:

○ NICU DAY # ____
○ HOME DAY # ____

## Today We Got To

☐ PHONE CALL    ☐ SKIN TO SKIN    ☐ SING
☐ TOUCH         ☐ TAKE TEMP       ☐ BATH
☐ DIAPER        ☐ FEEDING         ☐ MASSAGE
☐ HOLD          ☐ READ            ☐ VISITORS

☐ PHONE CALL    ☐ SKIN TO SKIN    ☐ SING
☐ TOUCH         ☐ TAKE TEMP       ☐ BATH
☐ DIAPER        ☐ FEEDING         ☐ MASSAGE
☐ HOLD          ☐ READ            ☐ VISITORS

## Feedings

_____    _____
_____    _____
_____    _____
_____    _____
_____    _____
_____    _____
_____    _____
_____    _____

## Medical Stats

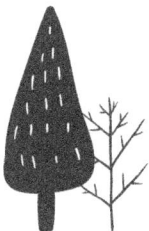
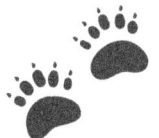

# Journaling

_____

_____

_____

_____

_____

_____

_____

_____

_____

_____

_____

_____

_____

_____

_____

_____

_____

_____

## QUESTIONS
TO ASK

## Today I'm Grateful For...

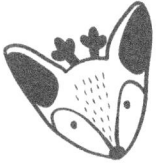
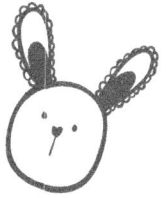

DATE:

_____   NAME                    _____   NAME

○ NICU DAY # ____    GESTATIONAL AGE:        GESTATIONAL AGE:        ○ NICU DAY # ____
○ HOME DAY # ____    WEIGHT:                 WEIGHT:                 ○ HOME DAY # ____

## Today We Got To

☐ PHONE CALL   ☐ SKIN TO SKIN   ☐ SING       ☐ PHONE CALL   ☐ SKIN TO SKIN   ☐ SING
☐ TOUCH        ☐ TAKE TEMP      ☐ BATH       ☐ TOUCH        ☐ TAKE TEMP      ☐ BATH
☐ DIAPER       ☐ FEEDING        ☐ MASSAGE    ☐ DIAPER       ☐ FEEDING        ☐ MASSAGE
☐ HOLD         ☐ READ           ☐ VISITORS   ☐ HOLD         ☐ READ           ☐ VISITORS

## Feedings

_____                    _____
_____                    _____
_____                    _____
_____                    _____
_____                    _____
_____                    _____
_____                    _____
_____                    _____

## Medical Stats

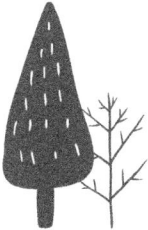
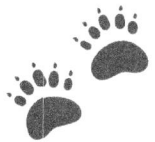

# Journaling

QUESTIONS
TO ASK

Today I'm Grateful For...

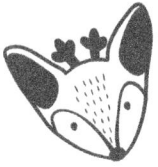
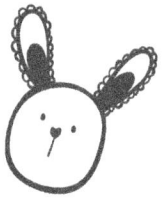

DATE:

_____ NAME

_____ NAME

○ NICU DAY # ____
○ HOME DAY # ____

GESTATIONAL AGE:

WEIGHT:

GESTATIONAL AGE:

WEIGHT:

○ NICU DAY # ____
○ HOME DAY # ____

## Today We Got To

☐ PHONE CALL    ☐ SKIN TO SKIN    ☐ SING
☐ TOUCH         ☐ TAKE TEMP       ☐ BATH
☐ DIAPER        ☐ FEEDING         ☐ MASSAGE
☐ HOLD          ☐ READ            ☐ VISITORS

☐ PHONE CALL    ☐ SKIN TO SKIN    ☐ SING
☐ TOUCH         ☐ TAKE TEMP       ☐ BATH
☐ DIAPER        ☐ FEEDING         ☐ MASSAGE
☐ HOLD          ☐ READ            ☐ VISITORS

## Feedings

_____     _____
_____     _____
_____     _____
_____     _____
_____     _____
_____     _____
_____     _____
_____     _____

## Medical Stats

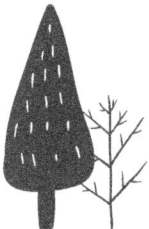
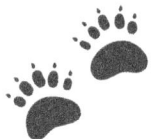

# Journaling

_____
_____
_____
_____
_____
_____
_____
_____
_____
_____
_____
_____
_____
_____
_____
_____
_____
_____
_____

QUESTIONS
TO ASK

Today I'm Grateful For...

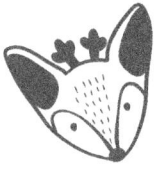
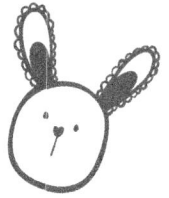

DATE:

_____ NAME

NAME _____

○ NICU DAY # _____
○ HOME DAY # _____

GESTATIONAL AGE:

WEIGHT:

GESTATIONAL AGE:

WEIGHT:

○ NICU DAY # _____
○ HOME DAY # _____

## Today We Got To

☐ PHONE CALL     ☐ SKIN TO SKIN     ☐ SING
☐ TOUCH          ☐ TAKE TEMP        ☐ BATH
☐ DIAPER         ☐ FEEDING          ☐ MASSAGE
☐ HOLD           ☐ READ             ☐ VISITORS

☐ PHONE CALL     ☐ SKIN TO SKIN     ☐ SING
☐ TOUCH          ☐ TAKE TEMP        ☐ BATH
☐ DIAPER         ☐ FEEDING          ☐ MASSAGE
☐ HOLD           ☐ READ             ☐ VISITORS

## Feedings

_____        _____
_____        _____
_____        _____
_____        _____
_____        _____
_____        _____
_____        _____
_____        _____

## Medical Stats

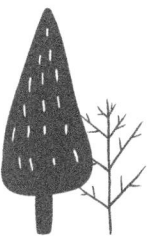
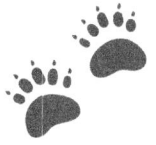

# Journaling

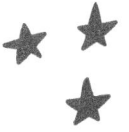

_____
_____
_____
_____
_____
_____
_____
_____
_____
_____
_____
_____
_____
_____
_____
_____
_____
_____
_____

## QUESTIONS
### TO ASK

Today I'm Grateful For...

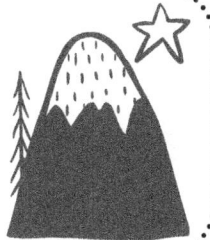

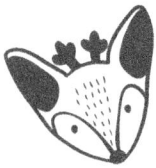
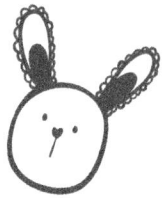

DATE:

_____                    _____
NAME                                          NAME

○ NICU DAY # ____    ┌─────────────────┐   ┌─────────────────┐   ○ NICU DAY # ____
○ HOME DAY # ____    │ GESTATIONAL AGE:│   │ GESTATIONAL AGE:│   ○ HOME DAY # ____
                     │                 │   │                 │
                     │ WEIGHT:         │   │ WEIGHT:         │
                     └─────────────────┘   └─────────────────┘

## Today We Got To

☐ PHONE CALL   ☐ SKIN TO SKIN   ☐ SING       ☐ PHONE CALL   ☐ SKIN TO SKIN   ☐ SING
☐ TOUCH        ☐ TAKE TEMP      ☐ BATH       ☐ TOUCH        ☐ TAKE TEMP      ☐ BATH
☐ DIAPER       ☐ FEEDING        ☐ MASSAGE    ☐ DIAPER       ☐ FEEDING        ☐ MASSAGE
☐ HOLD         ☐ READ           ☐ VISITORS   ☐ HOLD         ☐ READ           ☐ VISITORS

## Feedings

_____                    _____
_____                    _____
_____                    _____
_____                    _____
_____                    _____
_____                    _____
_____                    _____
_____                    _____

## Medical Stats

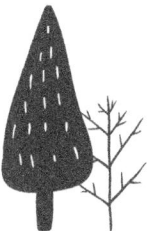
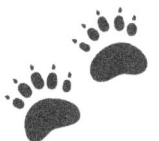

# Journaling

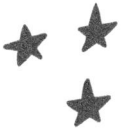

_____
_____
_____
_____
_____
_____
_____
_____
_____
_____
_____
_____
_____

## QUESTIONS
### TO ASK

_____
_____
_____
_____

### Today I'm Grateful For...

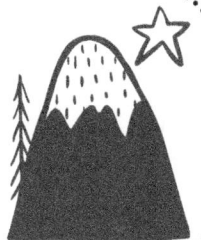

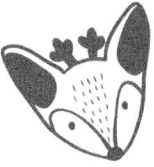

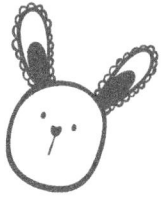

DATE:

_____
NAME

_____
NAME

○ NICU DAY # ____
○ HOME DAY # ____

GESTATIONAL AGE:

WEIGHT:

GESTATIONAL AGE:

WEIGHT:

○ NICU DAY # ____
○ HOME DAY # ____

## Today We Got To

☐ PHONE CALL    ☐ SKIN TO SKIN    ☐ SING
☐ TOUCH         ☐ TAKE TEMP       ☐ BATH
☐ DIAPER        ☐ FEEDING         ☐ MASSAGE
☐ HOLD          ☐ READ            ☐ VISITORS

☐ PHONE CALL    ☐ SKIN TO SKIN    ☐ SING
☐ TOUCH         ☐ TAKE TEMP       ☐ BATH
☐ DIAPER        ☐ FEEDING         ☐ MASSAGE
☐ HOLD          ☐ READ            ☐ VISITORS

## Feedings

## Medical Stats

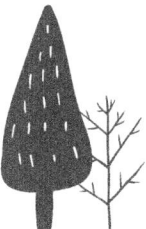

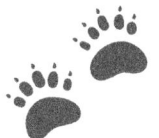

# Journaling

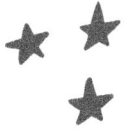

_____

_____

_____

_____

_____

_____

_____

_____

_____

_____

_____

_____

_____

_____

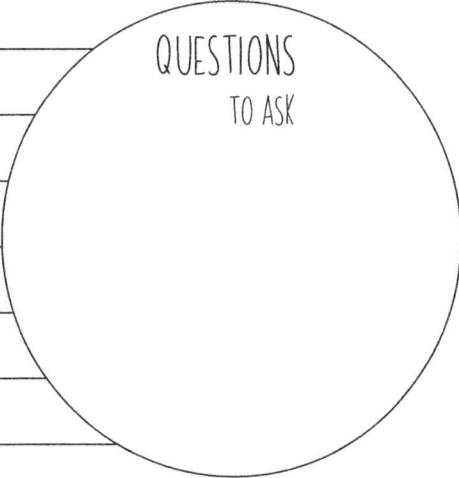

## QUESTIONS
### TO ASK

Today I'm Grateful For...

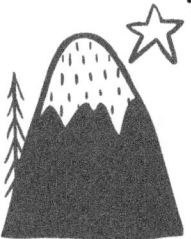

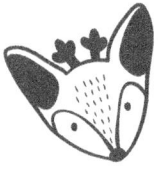
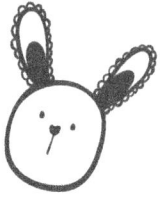

DATE:

_____ NAME

NAME _____

○ NICU DAY # ____
○ HOME DAY # ____

GESTATIONAL AGE:

WEIGHT:

GESTATIONAL AGE:

WEIGHT:

○ NICU DAY # ____
○ HOME DAY # ____

## Today We Got To

☐ PHONE CALL
☐ TOUCH
☐ DIAPER
☐ HOLD

☐ SKIN TO SKIN
☐ TAKE TEMP
☐ FEEDING
☐ READ

☐ SING
☐ BATH
☐ MASSAGE
☐ VISITORS

☐ PHONE CALL
☐ TOUCH
☐ DIAPER
☐ HOLD

☐ SKIN TO SKIN
☐ TAKE TEMP
☐ FEEDING
☐ READ

☐ SING
☐ BATH
☐ MASSAGE
☐ VISITORS

## Feedings

## Medical Stats

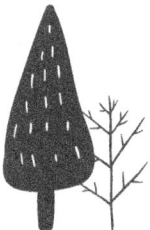
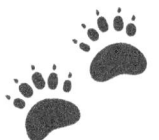

# Journaling

QUESTIONS
TO ASK

Today I'm Grateful For...

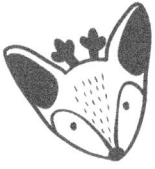
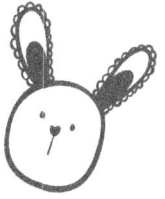

DATE:

_____ NAME

_____ NAME

○ NICU DAY # ____
○ HOME DAY # ____

GESTATIONAL AGE:

WEIGHT:

GESTATIONAL AGE:

WEIGHT:

○ NICU DAY # ____
○ HOME DAY # ____

## Today We Got To

☐ PHONE CALL   ☐ SKIN TO SKIN   ☐ SING
☐ TOUCH        ☐ TAKE TEMP      ☐ BATH
☐ DIAPER       ☐ FEEDING        ☐ MASSAGE
☐ HOLD         ☐ READ           ☐ VISITORS

☐ PHONE CALL   ☐ SKIN TO SKIN   ☐ SING
☐ TOUCH        ☐ TAKE TEMP      ☐ BATH
☐ DIAPER       ☐ FEEDING        ☐ MASSAGE
☐ HOLD         ☐ READ           ☐ VISITORS

## Feedings

_____     _____
_____     _____
_____     _____
_____     _____
_____     _____
_____     _____
_____     _____
_____     _____

## Medical Stats

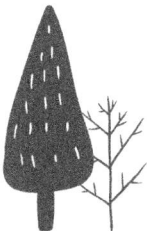
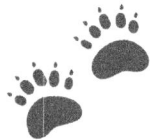

# Journaling

_____
_____
_____
_____
_____
_____
_____
_____
_____
_____
_____
_____
_____
_____
_____
_____
_____
_____
_____

## QUESTIONS
### TO ASK

Today I'm Grateful For...

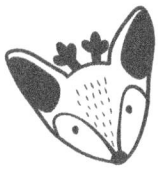

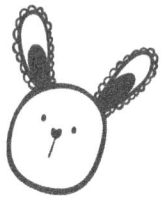

## DATE:

_____ NAME

_____ NAME

○ NICU DAY # ____
○ HOME DAY # ____

GESTATIONAL AGE:

WEIGHT:

GESTATIONAL AGE:

WEIGHT:

○ NICU DAY # ____
○ HOME DAY # ____

## Today We Got To

☐ PHONE CALL   ☐ SKIN TO SKIN   ☐ SING
☐ TOUCH        ☐ TAKE TEMP      ☐ BATH
☐ DIAPER       ☐ FEEDING        ☐ MASSAGE
☐ HOLD         ☐ READ           ☐ VISITORS

☐ PHONE CALL   ☐ SKIN TO SKIN   ☐ SING
☐ TOUCH        ☐ TAKE TEMP      ☐ BATH
☐ DIAPER       ☐ FEEDING        ☐ MASSAGE
☐ HOLD         ☐ READ           ☐ VISITORS

## Feedings

_____
_____
_____
_____
_____
_____
_____
_____
_____

_____
_____
_____
_____
_____
_____
_____
_____

## Medical Stats

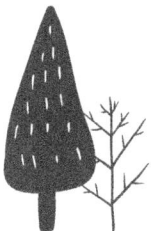

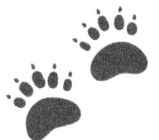

# Journaling

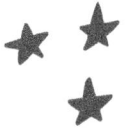

_____
_____
_____
_____
_____
_____
_____
_____
_____
_____
_____
_____
_____
_____
_____

## QUESTIONS
TO ASK

_____
_____
_____
_____
_____

Today I'm Grateful For...

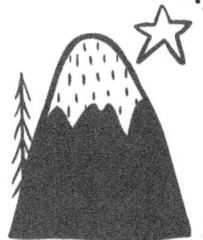

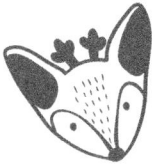
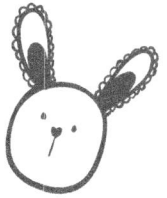

DATE:

NAME

NAME

○ NICU DAY # ____
○ HOME DAY # ____

GESTATIONAL AGE:

WEIGHT:

GESTATIONAL AGE:

WEIGHT:

○ NICU DAY # ____
○ HOME DAY # ____

## Today We Got To

☐ PHONE CALL
☐ TOUCH
☐ DIAPER
☐ HOLD

☐ SKIN TO SKIN
☐ TAKE TEMP
☐ FEEDING
☐ READ

☐ SING
☐ BATH
☐ MASSAGE
☐ VISITORS

☐ PHONE CALL
☐ TOUCH
☐ DIAPER
☐ HOLD

☐ SKIN TO SKIN
☐ TAKE TEMP
☐ FEEDING
☐ READ

☐ SING
☐ BATH
☐ MASSAGE
☐ VISITORS

## Feedings

## Medical Stats

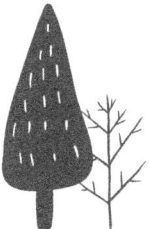
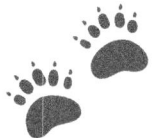

# Journaling

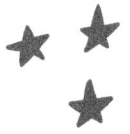

_____

_____

_____

_____

_____

_____

_____

_____

_____

_____

_____

_____

_____

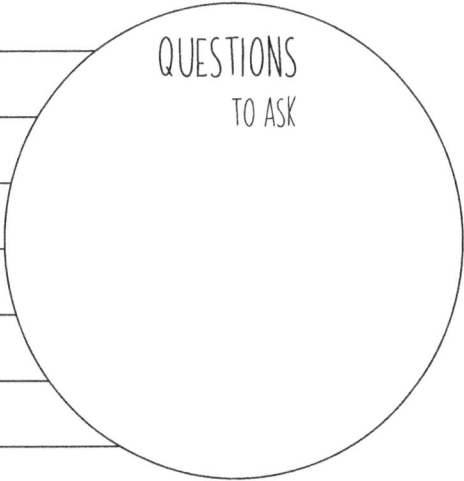

QUESTIONS
TO ASK

_____

_____

_____

_____

_____

Today I'm Grateful For...

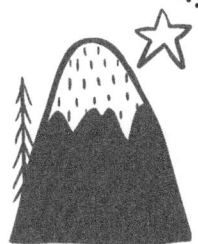

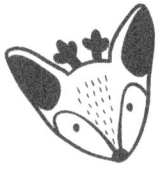
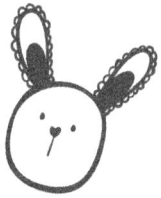

DATE:

_____  _____
NAME                      NAME

○ NICU DAY # ____
○ HOME DAY # ____

GESTATIONAL AGE:

WEIGHT:

GESTATIONAL AGE:

WEIGHT:

○ NICU DAY # ____
○ HOME DAY # ____

## Today We Got To

☐ PHONE CALL     ☐ SKIN TO SKIN     ☐ SING
☐ TOUCH          ☐ TAKE TEMP        ☐ BATH
☐ DIAPER         ☐ FEEDING          ☐ MASSAGE
☐ HOLD           ☐ READ             ☐ VISITORS

☐ PHONE CALL     ☐ SKIN TO SKIN     ☐ SING
☐ TOUCH          ☐ TAKE TEMP        ☐ BATH
☐ DIAPER         ☐ FEEDING          ☐ MASSAGE
☐ HOLD           ☐ READ             ☐ VISITORS

## Feedings

_____
_____
_____
_____
_____
_____
_____
_____

_____
_____
_____
_____
_____
_____
_____
_____

## Medical Stats

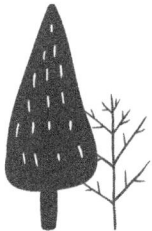
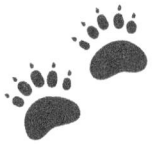

# Journaling

_____

_____

_____

_____

_____

_____

_____

_____

_____

_____

_____

_____

_____

## QUESTIONS
### TO ASK

_____

_____

_____

_____

_____

Today I'm Grateful For...

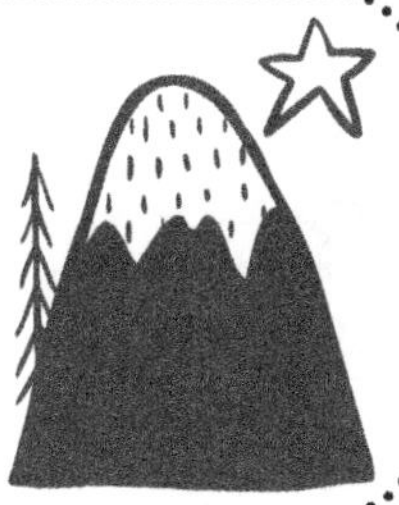

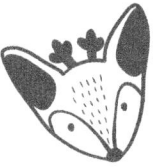

# DATE:

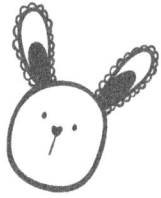

_____ NAME

NAME _____

○ NICU DAY # ____
○ HOME DAY # ____

GESTATIONAL AGE:

WEIGHT:

GESTATIONAL AGE:

WEIGHT:

○ NICU DAY # ____
○ HOME DAY # ____

## Today We Got To

☐ PHONE CALL   ☐ SKIN TO SKIN   ☐ SING
☐ TOUCH        ☐ TAKE TEMP      ☐ BATH
☐ DIAPER       ☐ FEEDING        ☐ MASSAGE
☐ HOLD         ☐ READ           ☐ VISITORS

☐ PHONE CALL   ☐ SKIN TO SKIN   ☐ SING
☐ TOUCH        ☐ TAKE TEMP      ☐ BATH
☐ DIAPER       ☐ FEEDING        ☐ MASSAGE
☐ HOLD         ☐ READ           ☐ VISITORS

## Feedings

_____
_____
_____
_____
_____
_____
_____
_____

_____
_____
_____
_____
_____
_____
_____
_____

## Medical Stats

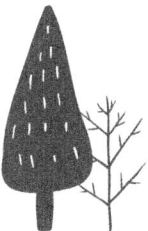

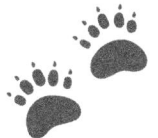

# Journaling

_____
_____
_____
_____
_____
_____
_____
_____
_____
_____
_____
_____

QUESTIONS
TO ASK

_____
_____
_____
_____
_____

Today I'm Grateful For...

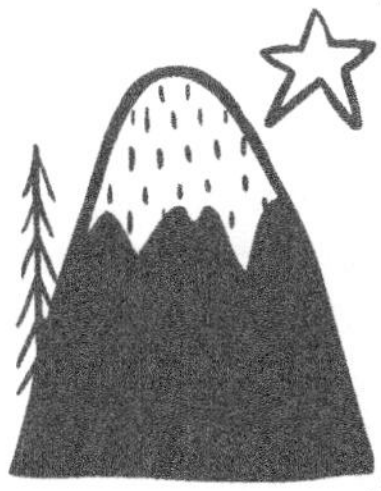

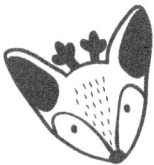
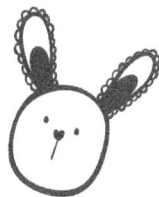

## DATE:

_____ NAME

NAME _____

○ NICU DAY # ____
○ HOME DAY # ____

GESTATIONAL AGE:

WEIGHT:

GESTATIONAL AGE:

WEIGHT:

○ NICU DAY # ____
○ HOME DAY # ____

## Today We Got To

☐ PHONE CALL   ☐ SKIN TO SKIN   ☐ SING
☐ TOUCH        ☐ TAKE TEMP      ☐ BATH
☐ DIAPER       ☐ FEEDING        ☐ MASSAGE
☐ HOLD         ☐ READ           ☐ VISITORS

☐ PHONE CALL   ☐ SKIN TO SKIN   ☐ SING
☐ TOUCH        ☐ TAKE TEMP      ☐ BATH
☐ DIAPER       ☐ FEEDING        ☐ MASSAGE
☐ HOLD         ☐ READ           ☐ VISITORS

## Feedings

## Medical Stats

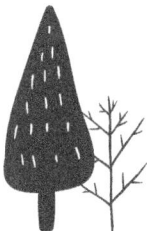
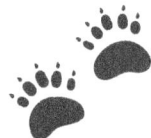

# Journaling

_____
_____
_____
_____
_____
_____
_____
_____
_____
_____
_____
_____
_____
_____
_____
_____

QUESTIONS
TO ASK

Today I'm Grateful For...

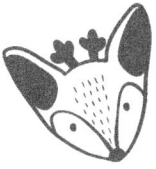
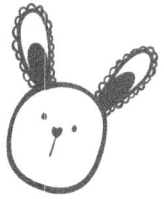

DATE:

_____ NAME

_____ NAME

○ NICU DAY # ____
○ HOME DAY # ____

GESTATIONAL AGE:

WEIGHT:

GESTATIONAL AGE:

WEIGHT:

○ NICU DAY # ____
○ HOME DAY # ____

## Today We Got To

☐ PHONE CALL    ☐ SKIN TO SKIN    ☐ SING
☐ TOUCH         ☐ TAKE TEMP       ☐ BATH
☐ DIAPER        ☐ FEEDING         ☐ MASSAGE
☐ HOLD          ☐ READ            ☐ VISITORS

☐ PHONE CALL    ☐ SKIN TO SKIN    ☐ SING
☐ TOUCH         ☐ TAKE TEMP       ☐ BATH
☐ DIAPER        ☐ FEEDING         ☐ MASSAGE
☐ HOLD          ☐ READ            ☐ VISITORS

## Feedings

_____        _____
_____        _____
_____        _____
_____        _____
_____        _____
_____        _____
_____        _____
_____        _____

## Medical Stats

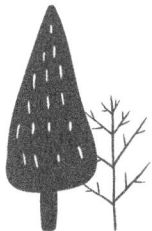
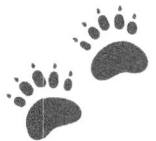

# Journaling

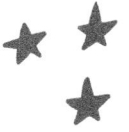

_____
_____
_____
_____
_____
_____
_____
_____
_____
_____
_____
_____
_____
_____
_____
_____
_____
_____
_____

## QUESTIONS
### TO ASK

Today I'm Grateful For...

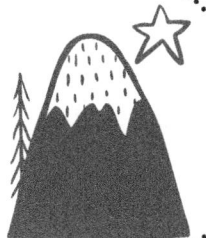

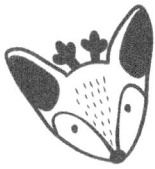
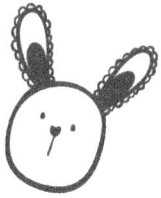

| DATE: |
|-------|

_____  NAME  _____  NAME

○ NICU DAY # ____
○ HOME DAY # ____

| GESTATIONAL AGE: | GESTATIONAL AGE: |
| WEIGHT: | WEIGHT: |

○ NICU DAY # ____
○ HOME DAY # ____

## Today We Got To

☐ PHONE CALL   ☐ SKIN TO SKIN   ☐ SING
☐ TOUCH        ☐ TAKE TEMP       ☐ BATH
☐ DIAPER       ☐ FEEDING         ☐ MASSAGE
☐ HOLD         ☐ READ            ☐ VISITORS

☐ PHONE CALL   ☐ SKIN TO SKIN   ☐ SING
☐ TOUCH        ☐ TAKE TEMP       ☐ BATH
☐ DIAPER       ☐ FEEDING         ☐ MASSAGE
☐ HOLD         ☐ READ            ☐ VISITORS

## Feedings

_____
_____
_____
_____
_____
_____
_____
_____

_____
_____
_____
_____
_____
_____
_____
_____

## Medical Stats

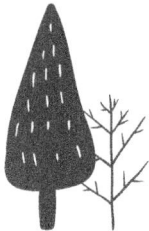
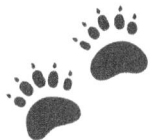

# Journaling

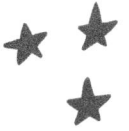

## QUESTIONS
TO ASK

Today I'm Grateful For...

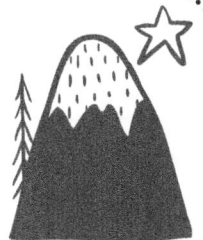

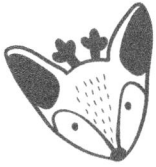
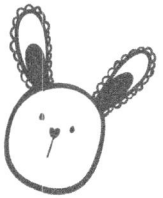

DATE:

NAME

NAME

○ NICU DAY # ____
○ HOME DAY # ____

GESTATIONAL AGE:

WEIGHT:

GESTATIONAL AGE:

WEIGHT:

○ NICU DAY # ____
○ HOME DAY # ____

## Today We Got To

☐ PHONE CALL
☐ TOUCH
☐ DIAPER
☐ HOLD

☐ SKIN TO SKIN
☐ TAKE TEMP
☐ FEEDING
☐ READ

☐ SING
☐ BATH
☐ MASSAGE
☐ VISITORS

☐ PHONE CALL
☐ TOUCH
☐ DIAPER
☐ HOLD

☐ SKIN TO SKIN
☐ TAKE TEMP
☐ FEEDING
☐ READ

☐ SING
☐ BATH
☐ MASSAGE
☐ VISITORS

## Feedings

_____
_____
_____
_____
_____
_____
_____
_____

_____
_____
_____
_____
_____
_____
_____
_____

## Medical Stats

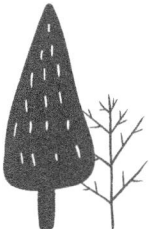
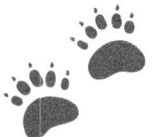

# Journaling

_____

_____

_____

_____

_____

_____

_____

_____

_____

_____

_____

_____

QUESTIONS
TO ASK

_____

_____

_____

_____

_____

Today I'm Grateful For...

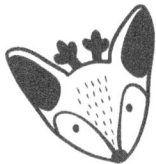
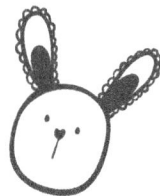

DATE:

_____
NAME

_____
NAME

○ NICU DAY # ____
○ HOME DAY # ____

GESTATIONAL AGE:

WEIGHT:

GESTATIONAL AGE:

WEIGHT:

○ NICU DAY # ____
○ HOME DAY # ____

## Today We Got To

☐ PHONE CALL  ☐ SKIN TO SKIN  ☐ SING
☐ TOUCH       ☐ TAKE TEMP     ☐ BATH
☐ DIAPER      ☐ FEEDING       ☐ MASSAGE
☐ HOLD        ☐ READ          ☐ VISITORS

☐ PHONE CALL  ☐ SKIN TO SKIN  ☐ SING
☐ TOUCH       ☐ TAKE TEMP     ☐ BATH
☐ DIAPER      ☐ FEEDING       ☐ MASSAGE
☐ HOLD        ☐ READ          ☐ VISITORS

## Feedings

_____
_____
_____
_____
_____
_____
_____
_____

_____
_____
_____
_____
_____
_____
_____
_____

## Medical Stats

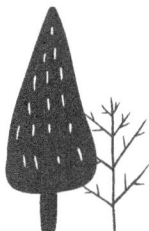
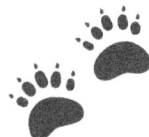

# Journaling

QUESTIONS
TO ASK

Today I'm Grateful For...

Made in the USA
Middletown, DE
28 April 2025

74884994R00104